A
Quick Cuppa
Herbal

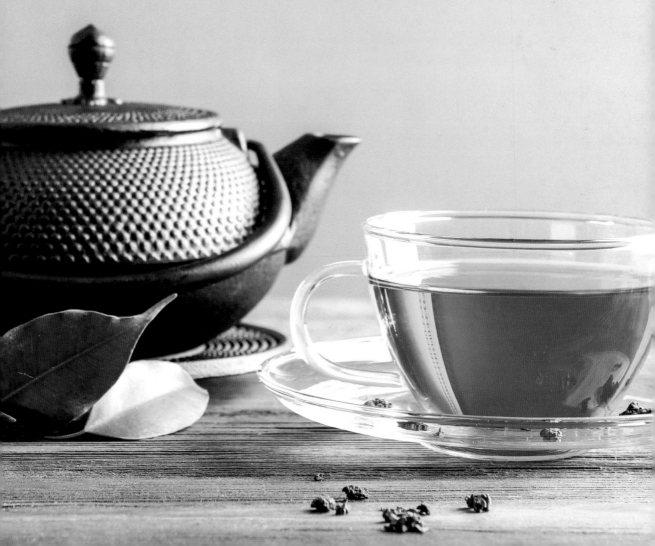

MERCIER PRESS
Cork
www.mercierpress.ie

© Fiann Ó Nualláin, 2019
Photography © Adobe Stock

ISBN: 978 1 78117 670 2

A CIP record for this title is available from the British Library.

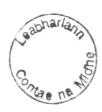

Printed and bound in the EU.

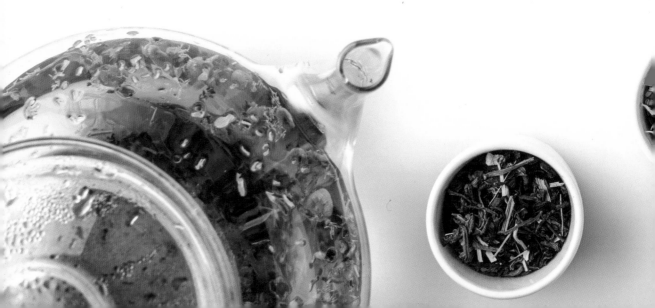

A Quick Cuppa Herbal

Fiann Ó Nualláin

The
Holistic
Gardener

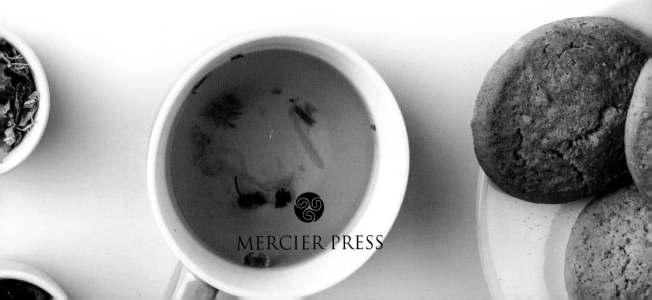

MERCIER PRESS

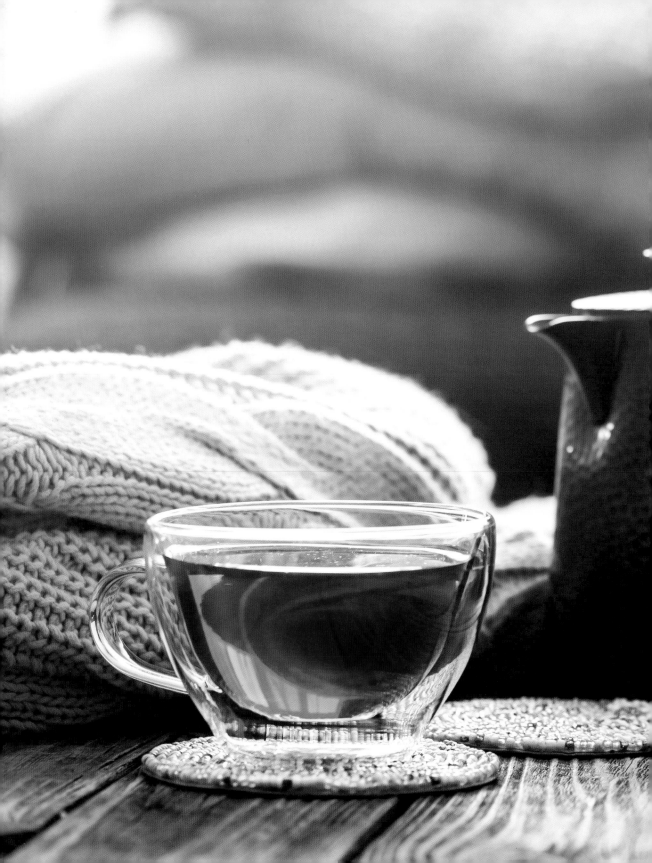

'Tea is the ultimate mental and medical remedy and has the ability to make one's life more full and complete.'

Myōan Eisai - from *Kissa Yojoki,*
aka 'How to Stay Healthy by Drinking Tea'

circa AD 1211

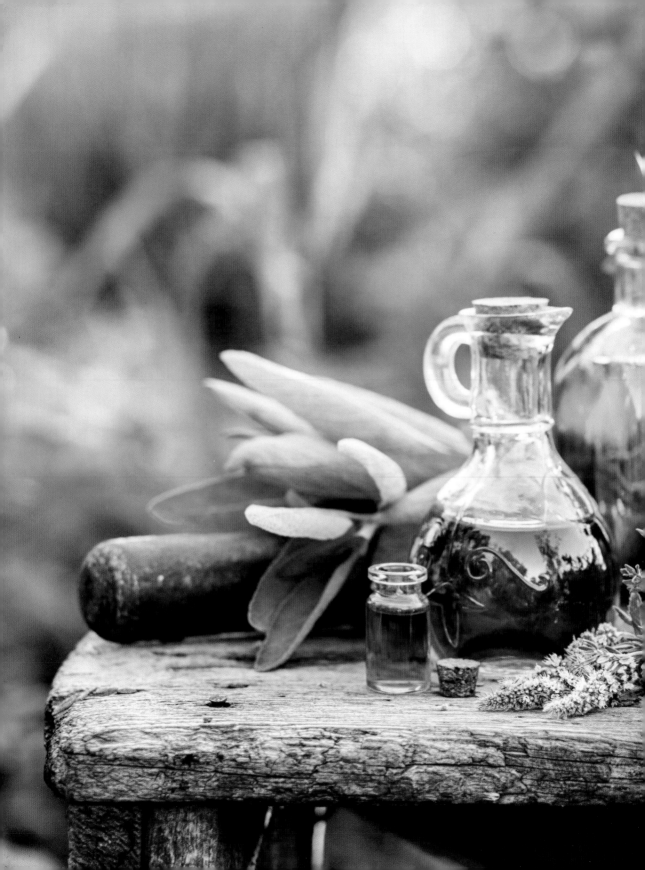

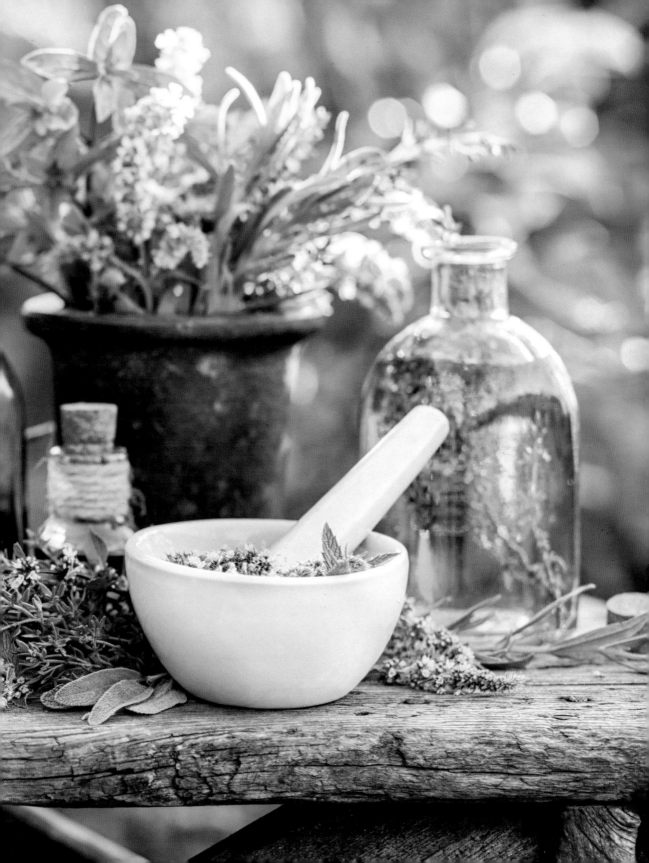

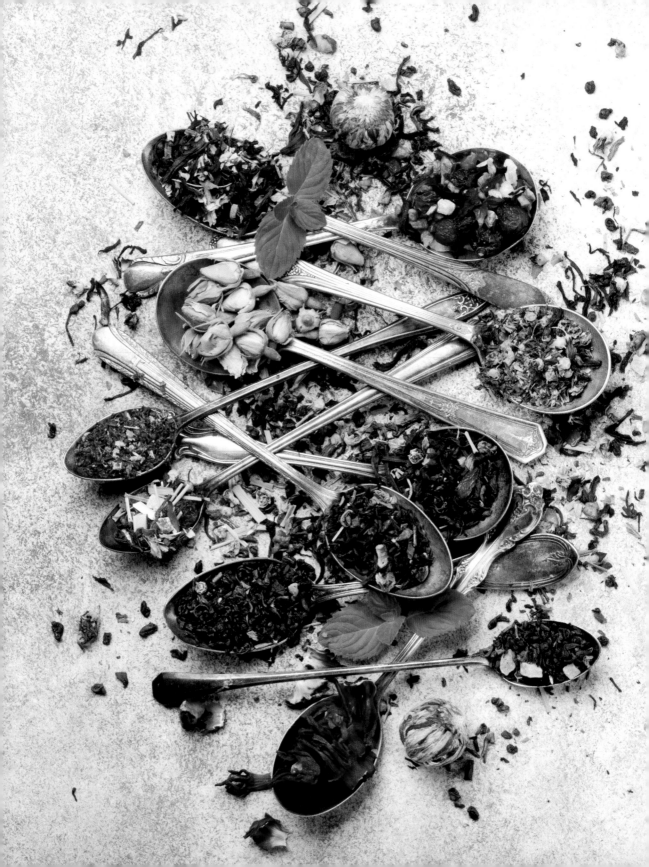

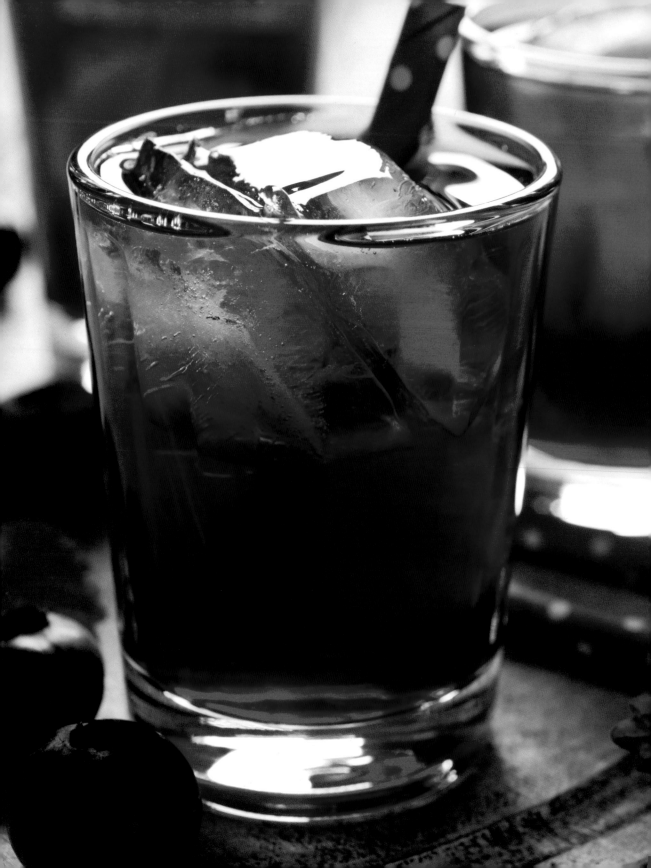

Introduction

'Drinking a daily cup of tea will surely
starve the apothecary.'

Chinese Proverb

In the modern world of 'health consciousness', herbal teas are all the rage: as a low- or no-caffeine alternative to regular tea or coffee, as a beverage with benefits, or simply as a nod to the intention of being well and considerate of our bodies. But with so much choice in herbal teas, do we actually know what we are drinking? Sure it's a healthy alternative to carbonated, caffeinated or sugar-loaded beverages, but it is also a herb and herbs carry medicinal weight. So what is the medicine in a cup of rosehip tea and what good might hibiscus or lemon balm tea do you? When should you avoid mint tea or reach for the nettle? What are we actually drinking? What are the pros and cons?

For some herbal tea drinkers, a glossy magazine article or morning TV show may have provided some basic information, so they reach for the peppermint tea to ease their digestive upset, while others may be on the valerian to combat a recent bout of insomnia. For these people, the herbal tea is not just a healthier beverage choice, it is the medicine for their current health problem. The issue with this, however, is that the basic information provided may not have included advice on important aspects such as dosage or contraindications (reasons not to drink a certain tea). Most proprietary brands don't even list on the packaging what the properties or medicinal actions of the tea may be. This book aims to address that.

It explores sixty of the most popular and easily accessible herbal teas – those readily found on the shelves of supermarkets, local shops or the nearest health store, as well as a few you can harvest from the garden or spice rack. It explains some of their potential uses or inherent medicinal chemistry, and is compiled in a similar way to a 'herbal' or materia medica. The book is called *A Quick Cuppa Herbal* because of this 'herbal' construct and because a quick cup of plant medicine is not just a great way to gain the medicinal actions of the plant's chemistry, but is also the handiest method of home herbalism.

Increasingly people are turning to home herbalism to meet their health needs, and while snappy apps and Google searches may potentially enlighten, my background in medicinal botany means I approach this with a degree of expertise that can cut to the point and filter the accurate facts from those so-called 'health statements' reported as matter of fact. Extensive research has gone into honing this book to a correct, precise and accessible read, and all medical facts herein have been rigorously validated by scientific study – many of those studies are listed in the bibliography.

The goodness in these herbal teas is viewed through the lens of their traditional uses (some extending back hundreds of years, while others have been in use for thousands of years) and also with the insight of some modern science to explore exactly why they have stood the test of time and what actions they utilise to be all-round health promoting.

To address herbal tea in the context of its healing potential, and not just as a caffeine alternative, I have detailed the medicinal applications of each tea and also explored the potential of that tea as a therapeutic agent in illness treatment and health management, with dosage and cautions included. However, to be clear: this is not a self-medication manual, as no book can take your individual case history or any underlying conditions unique to you into consideration. What the book can do, in promoting a fuller understanding of the medicinal actions and consumption parameters of each tea listed, is help you make a more informed choice when next in the herbal tea aisle or selecting today's lunchtime brew. If you wish to apply the knowledge contained within these pages to an ongoing serious health issue, however, then I would advise that you also consult a health professional who can supervise and guide a holistic approach to resolving that issue. Thereafter, there will be plenty of time to starve the apothecary.

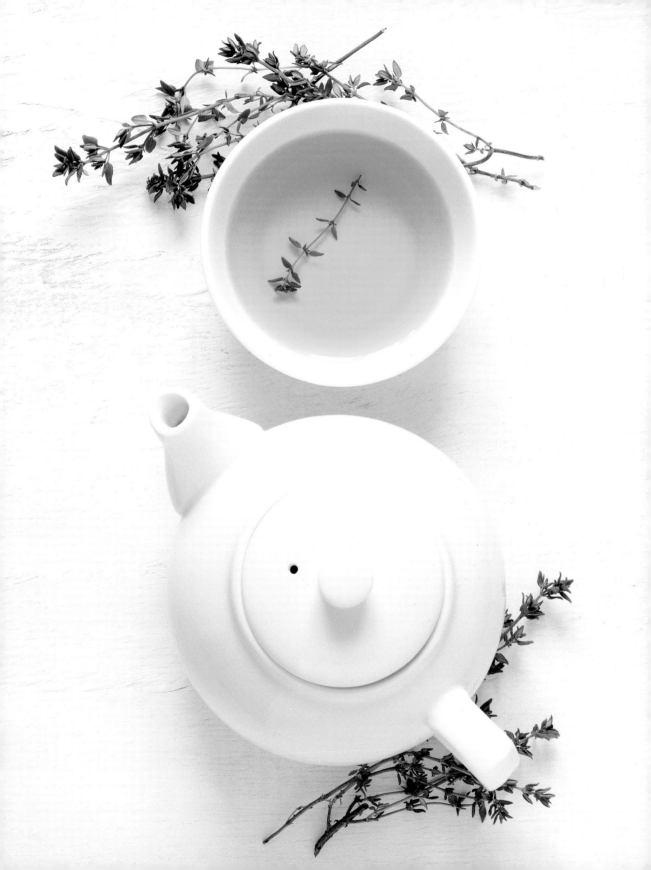

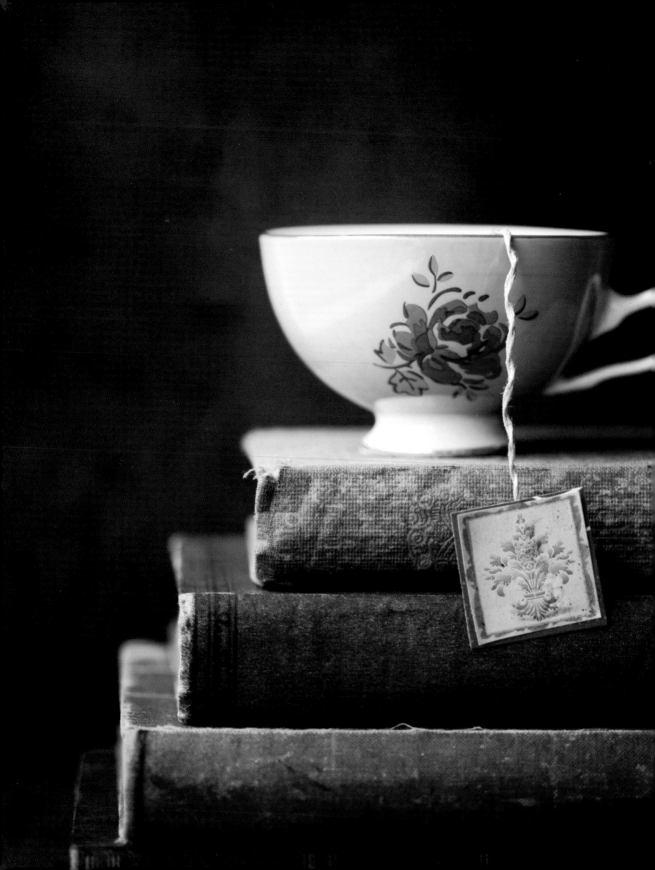

A Fortuitous Wind: The Invention of Tea

While this book is all about herbal teas, I have also included an entry on what some people call 'true tea' (*Camellia sinensis*) in the form of green tea. I have done this because green tea is often found unadulterated on the herbal tea shelf and also as a herbal blend – mixed with herbs and extracts to extend its unique healing profile. True tea is perhaps the very inspiration of herbalism, i.e. the origin of the idea of taking a plant part and using hot water to extract its beneficial chemistry into an easily replicated beverage form.

Legend has it that the Chinese emperor known as Shen Nong (*circa* 2737 BC) favoured his drinking water hot. One day, while he was having his midday beverage outside in the garden near his palace's prize camellia bushes, a wind rose up and blew a leaf into his cup, and so alluring was the aroma emitted from the hot cup that the emperor decided not to discard but to taste. The pleasantness of the sip enticed another, and on completion of the beverage he felt refreshed and enlivened and decided to replicate the event for his next quenching of thirst. So began a daily routine, one which was soon replicated by his courtiers, and thus a tradition was born that would soon reach beyond the palace walls and tempt the whole world.

In other versions of the legend, the emperor, inspired by the energy-gifting camellia leaf, went on to explore other leaves and plant parts, and developed a medicinal knowledge through his experiments. There is, in the canon of early Chinese medical texts, a book known as *Shén Nóng Běnco Jīng*, aka *The Materia Medica of Shen Nong* (sometimes referred to as *The Divine Farmer's Classic of Materia Medica*). That book, really a collection of three treatises, is not only a herbal handbook, but also a study of sustainable agriculture and an exploration of natural science as well as spiritual life. It is an expression of the Chinese art of 'yǎng shēng' (nurturing life), which would in time inspire some aspects of Taoist philosophy and be embraced by Confucian and Buddhist teaching. It is nice to think of the 'three teachings' bonded and harmonised over a cup of tea.

So, from the start, tea was more than just a new brew found through serendipity; it was the fortuitous wind of inspiration that led to scientific exploration and an understanding of plants and their healing attributes. It was a new mechanism for the delivery of medicine.

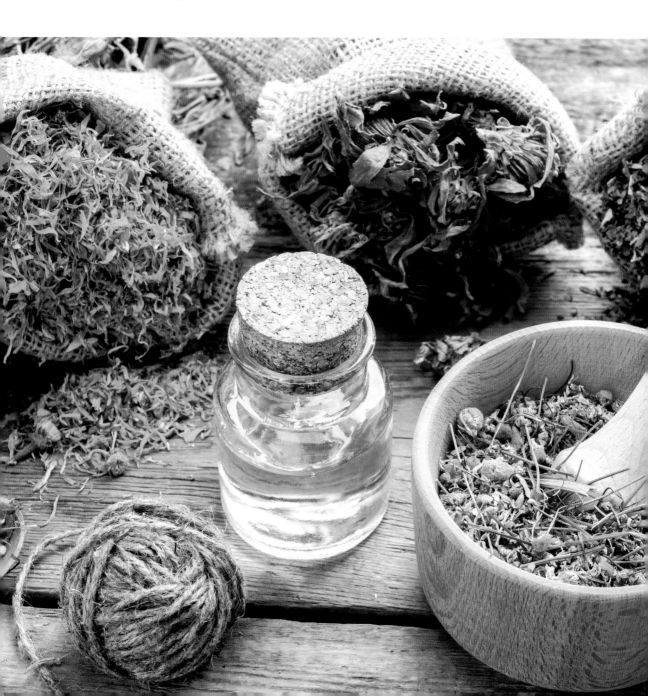

The Healthy Option

Herbal tea has become a byword for healthy. It is not just about what's *not* in it – herbal teas being generally caffeine free and drunk without milk or sugar – it is also about what *is* in it. All the plant constituents, from nutrients and minerals to antioxidant pigments and organic acids – scientifically referred to as phytochemicals – are active ingredients that facilitate the herbalism of the herb that yields the tea. So, for example, we now know that flavonoids – the natural compounds that provide colour to plant parts – can act as powerful antioxidants when taken into the human system and actually help protect our cells from oxidative stress (free radical damage), thereby slowing the ageing and deterioration process. Given that there is also a serious link between free radicals – unstable atoms formed within the body – and many chronic diseases and persistent illnesses, from fibromyalgia to dementia, it is clear that anything that prevents or eliminates them is a useful shot in the arm.

Some of the phytochemicals in these herbal teas are beneficial to both physical and mental/cognitive health, and are easily available to all. So, for example, Johnston (2015) notes that apigenin, found in chamomile, yarrow and passionflower (amongst others), is a flavone which acts on the brain and exerts a sedative and anxiety-reducing effect, effectively acting in a similar manner to many prescription anti-anxiety medications. On the physical health side, apigenin is also known to be an anticancer agent via its ability to trigger apoptosis and autophagy of damaged cells (basically, the death and clearance of cancerous cells), and, as the research of Xu (2008) and Yan (2017) shows, it can also induce cell cycle arrest, suppress cell migration and invasion, and stimulate a stronger immune response.

In this amped up, 24/7, modern world, physical responses to stress and the mental anxiety of perceived isolation, fear of missing out, status anxiety, etc., are driving a real crisis in personal well-being, productiveness potential and (dare I say it!) actually having a life. An instant digital detox would be to put the devices down, make a brew and sip it outside. If I may quote T'ien Yiheng, an eighth-century Chinese sage, 'Tea is drunk to forget the din of the world.'

We know many teas provide a physical detox, activating the liver or bile secretions to eliminate toxins. But tea is about more than that. Removing the din of the world is a spiritual tool and a cognitive detox for our troublesome or overexcited thought processes. The reality of sitting with a quick cup of herbal is perhaps especially relevant for those stuck in a negative thought process. In these cases, however, it is not just the gift of a time out, as there will be some beneficial phytochemistry at play too.

With depressed and irritated mood there is often a serotonin/vitamin-D deficiency at the root, just as there is a link between low blood levels of vitamin D and certain cancers. A dietary therapy of increased vitamin D is often proffered, but vitamin D is fat soluble and needs to be ingested with a fatty or oil content to be extracted digestively and absorbed efficiently. Apigenin, which acts in many of the same ways as vitamin D, is water-soluble and more easily absorbed from a herbal tea that contains it.

As you read on and into the individual entries in the tea directory, you will find that many of the teas listed impact directly upon brain chemistry and help improve our mood or advance increased cognitive function. For example, you will see that there are several phytochemicals that activate serotonin (the chemical neurotransmitter involved in our perception/experience of well-being and happiness), or switch off anxiety-released molecules. Many have sedative or nervine properties that calm the body and mind. Basically, the ones you love will love you back with a lift of the spirits every time you cherish the sip.

On days when you can't get your Zen on because the physical pain, the mental strain or the time drain of life's problems are tsunami strength, a cup of herbal tea is a care package of active medicine. Some of the more potent constituents found in plants, known as phenolic compounds, are also secondary metabolites. This means that they are active agents in plants, like an immune system contributing to botanical disease prevention – i.e. to stop plants getting mildew or viral infections. When these compounds are added to the human diet, they play an important role in maintaining human health – being antioxidant, anti-inflammatory and anticarcinogenic/antimutagenic. The role of phenolic compounds in cancer prevention has been extensively studied and they have been shown (Huang 2010, Luo 2004) to regulate both carcinogen metabolism and ontogenesis expression. It is noted (Shahidi 2000) that fruits, certain vegetables, herbal teas and herbal medicinal infusions are the chief contributors of phenolics to our diet.

In a fast-paced, fast food, quick lunch-break world, a cup of herbal tea may literally be a lifesaver, or at least an illness defender. For example, salicylic acid – the plant constituent that inspired the creation of aspirin (acetylsalicylic acid) – is a phenolic compound that suppresses pain perception. It is present in meadowsweet, blueberries and blackberries, amongst other things. Another example would be cannabinoids, the active constituents of cannabis, which are also phenolic compounds with pain-relieving action. The herbal and medicinal activities of echinacea, thyme, yarrow and St John's wort are the result of phenolic acid, notably caffeic and p-coumaric acids.

It is the good in the cup that each entry here will go on to explore. But before that, it would be good to explore some of the safety concerns around herbal teas.

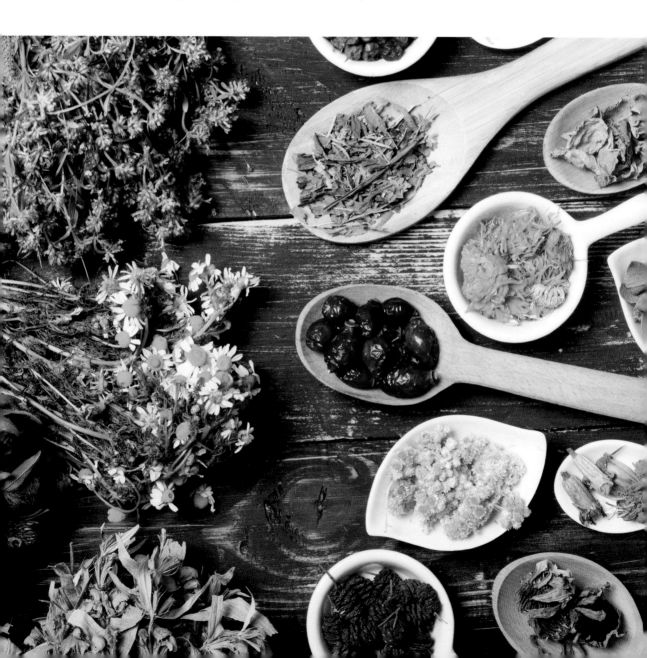

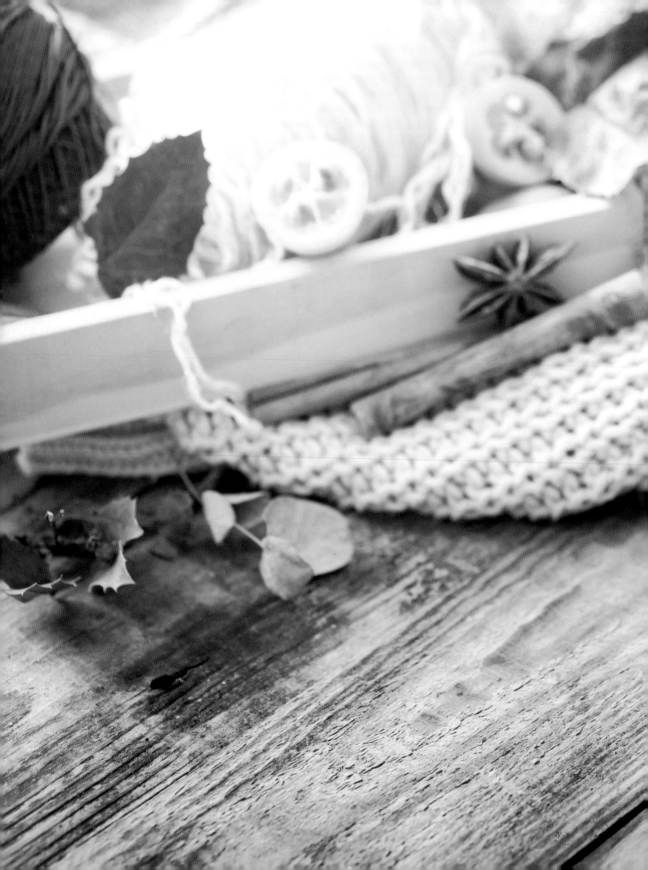

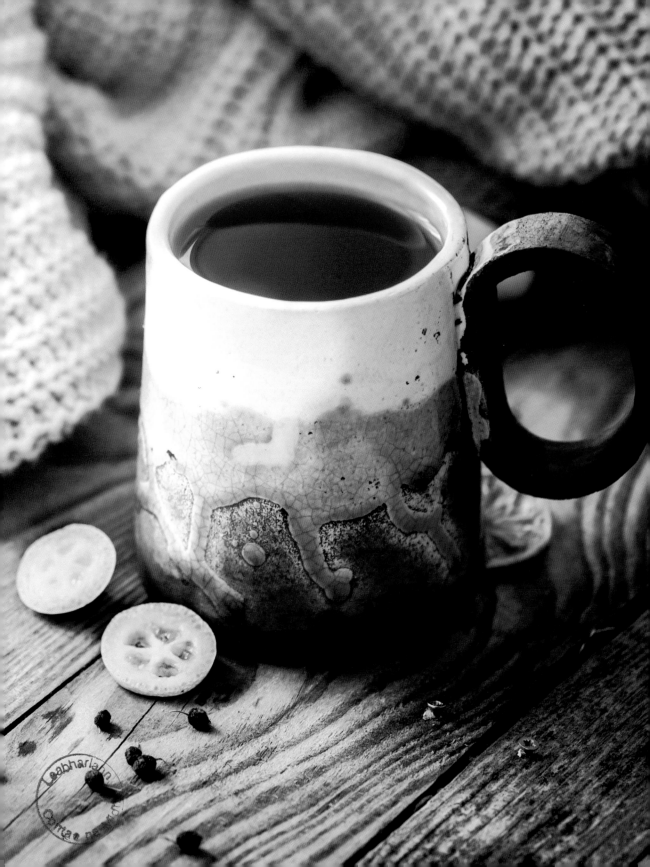

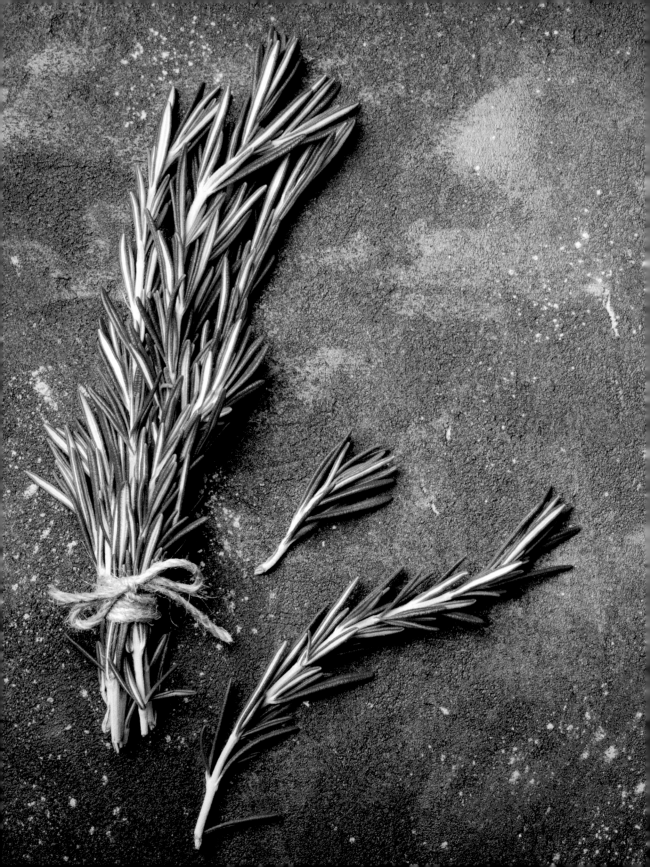

Safety Concerns

In an article titled 'Safety of Herbal v Orthodox Drugs' published in the *Irish Medical Times* in 2001, Paul McCarthy noted that 'Greater than 26,000 times more people die from preventable medical misadventure and properly regulated and controlled drugs than from herbal medicine.' There's a statistic you don't hear every day – and, yes, that by no means confirms that herbs are always the safest option for any particular condition or ailment, but it does answer some of the scaremongering around herbal medicine.

Herbs have been utilised in every age of human history. The oldest tombs and excavated graves reveal seeds and unguents of the ancients, many with plant parts still used today for everything from stomach upset to social diseases. As the saying goes – there is nothing new under the sun. In this timeline, foil-packed and patented pharmacology is but a blink of the eye. Of course, that does not mean go off your cancer or psychiatric meds for a week-long tea binge in expectation of a miracle cure. But might some teas support your treatment regime?

There are many who argue that the herbal option is more effective and for the vast population of the world more accessible and affordable than pharmaceuticals. Ekor (2013) notes that not less than 80 per cent of the world's population relies on traditional herbal medicines for some part of its primary healthcare. Herbal teas in our healing repertoire may be our future as well as our past.

The teas herein are all GRAS – generally regarded as safe. They do, however, have pharmacologically active components, so it is advisable to note the cautions in each entry and familiarise yourself with the wider context of the herb if you plan to use it medicinally or over extended periods. The main medicinal actions section is also a tip-off to potential contraindications – for example, if the herb is 'hypotensive', which means it will lower blood pressure, and you are already on hypotensive medication, then you may need to avoid this herb or at least seek further clarification from your health-care provider before trying it.

There is always the possibility of an allergic reaction to a phytoconstituent (component of the plant) previously not encountered, or a hidden action of a herb you had not suspected or known; there can also be some interaction with prescription medications and with conventional over-the-counter drugs (intensifying absorption, increasing the activity or cancelling out), and then there is the age-old question: 'Is it safe in pregnancy?' So let's address those issues now.

Adverse Reactions

Adverse reactions to herbal medicine can range from mild, allergic-type (e.g. hives) to severe (bronchial distress, anaphylactic shock). For the most part, however, the tick list of negative side effects (as ascribed often by opponents of herbal medicine) are headache, dizziness, dry mouth, nausea, vomiting, diarrhoea or constipation, restlessness or fatigue and, for some people, a bout of photosensitivity. But I dare you to read the leaflet that comes with your prescription medicine, or even an over-the-counter headache or travel sickness pill, and compare and contrast. The potential side effects of herbal medicine are slight in comparison.

That said, a side effect or adverse reaction is not only unpleasant, it is a 'do not' warning sign, as it means that this herb does not agree with you. Go off it immediately and think about a 'Plan B' in consultation with a health professional.

What's so good about a herbal tea is that you are not going to eat a kilo of a plant that you may be potentially allergic to; instead, you are going to imbibe a low dosage extract. Most adverse reactions to herbal medicines come from taking large dosages and from long-term or overuse. But as anyone can be allergic to anything, even in low dosage, it is always wise to be vigilant and ease yourself in. If you have taken the guidance of a professional, as previously advised, you should have less chance of any problems.

The thing is we don't know that we are allergic or sensitive to a chemical or phytochemical until we have the encounter. On the other hand, there may be glaring clues – say, if you are allergic to daisies and ragwort, then it seems likely that herbs in their botanical family may well trigger a reaction. That is why, in laying this book out as a more modern materia medica, I supply the botanical family names, as this will allow you to check for yourself where an issue might lie. Daisies and ragworts, for example, are in the Asteraceae (aka Compositae) family and so are artichoke, chicory and yarrow. Often the negative reaction – when there is one – is to the pollen and not the foliage, but this way you can exercise appropriate discretion and caution.

Drug Interactions

Sometimes herbal medicines make an ideal co-therapy to conventional medicine, but other times things can clash. Some phytochemicals can amplify the effects of prescription medications and so generate an undesirable reaction; other times a herb or food can interfere with the pharmacological efficiency of a prescribed drug, or the drug with the herb, and so limit or distort the healing potential and effectiveness of both.

Herbs that enhance the activity of gamma-aminobutyric acid (GABA) – a neurotransmitter that sends chemical messages through the brain and the nervous system – may similarly be overkill, or clash with antidepressant, anti-anxiety and tranquilliser medications. Some herbs thin blood and so would not be suitable if you are on blood thinners already. So if the medical actions listed are similar or counter to those of a prescription drug you are currently taking, then exercise due restraint and caution.

Tea and Pregnancy

Many women come to herbal tea as an alternative to caffeine beverages for the duration of their pregnancy and the first couple of months of breastfeeding. Caffeine can cross the placenta and enter the bloodstream of your unborn child, and can also enter breast milk in nursing mothers. Some women may have been alerted by a book, nutritionist, herbalist or health-care provider to some herbal teas that are beneficial in supporting well-being through pregnancy and also which may remedy pregnancy issues from indigestion to anxiety to strengthening the uterus.

However, all the usual cautions apply – if not a little more so – when consuming herbal teas during pregnancy and also during the following months, if breastfeeding. Some teas otherwise known to be safe, such as parsley or sage, are not recommended during or immediately after pregnancy as some of their medicinal actions can exert themselves on your unborn or breastfeeding child.

Then there are restrictions around any herb classed as an emmenagogue – i.e. herbs utilised to stimulate pelvic blood flow and uterus contractions. These are often used to bring on a delayed period, but can potentially (if misused by intent or dosage error) induce early labour. Some herbs have a milder emmenagogue effect, bringing about a raising of oestrogen levels, which can also stimulate pelvic blood flow. In the interest of safety all emmenagogue and oestrogenic potential will be identified in 'main medicinal actions'.

A lot of it is down to common sense, and the majority of herbal teas on the market are not imbided in quantities sufficient for complications. The fact is that there just is not sufficient study/research on the use of herbal teas during pregnancy and so the default of most advisory health organisations and most health providers is to play it safe and counsel avoidance or extremely limited exposure to herbal medicines in general.

In terms of a best practice, the consensus is not to exceed more than 4 cups of herbal tea per day during pregnancy and to change the variety of herbal tea that you consume each day, so that you are not reaching levels of medicinal dosage of one particular herb. It also helps to be aware of agents in food and herbs that can find their way into breast milk.

Even when it comes to the teas most recommended for pregnancy, do apply common sense and fuller research/consultation. Raspberry leaf, for example, has long been utilised to decrease nausea, tone the uterus, increase milk production and ease labour pains, but it is perhaps best not employed until the late second and the third trimester. Both ginger and peppermint teas are known to alleviate nausea and have a traditional usage with morning sickness and pregnancy digestive complaints, but they can prompt stronger heartburn in some.

Tea and Breastfeeding

Just as some women drink fennel or anise tea as a galactagogue (to increase milk supply), so, too, the phytochemicals of those plants make their way into the breast milk and are considered to be anti-colic to the receiving baby.

However, the potential of 'less useful' or 'potentially harmful' phytochemicals entering the infant via breast milk is a general cause for concern when it comes to cautions from doctors or forum groups, who therefore recommend against experimenting with herbs or supplements during pregnancy. Even green tea, with its lower caffeine content, is often on the banned list for the first five to six months of breastfeeding. From a cautionary viewpoint, strong medicinal herbs are best avoided during breastfeeding. Attention should also be drawn to the fact that some astringent herbs (blackberry, willow, yarrow, etc.) and teas with menthol (mint varieties) may inhibit milk flow.

Tea and Cancer Scares

Reports of tea consumption and higher risk of throat or mouth cancer is less about the herb and more about the temperature of the beverage. In 2016 the World Health Organization concluded that any hot beverage above 149°F (65°C) can contribute to an increased risk of oesophageal cancer. This is brought about by the repeated scald/burn of the hot tea causing damage, altering cellular structure and potentially triggering mutagenic changes. Yet in studies of high-temperature tea consumption and oesophageal cancer risk it has been disclosed that it was predominant amongst those who also engaged in alcohol and tobacco consumption. Conversely, many herbal teas and the potent antioxidants with green tea are often lauded as lowering cancer risk.

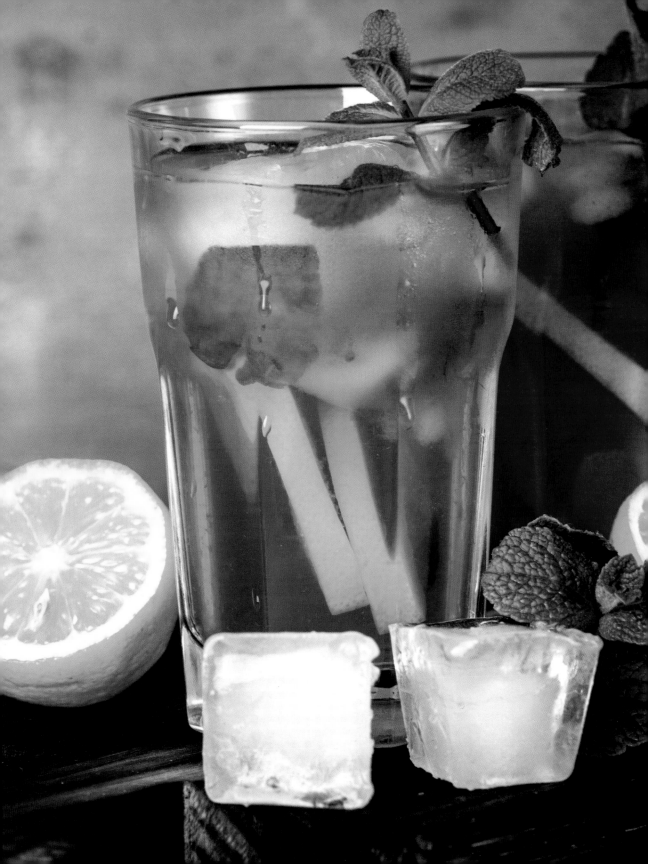

Correct Dosage

For the vast majority of herbal teas that are taken as a pleasant beverage with some knock-on health benefits, the consumption is often tied to meal times or morning and evening, and so generally would not exceed 2–3 cups per day. For the majority of herbal teas at a dosage of 1–2 teaspoons or 1 teabag, that range is considered safe. With more strongly therapeutic herbs, such as those that may lower blood pressure or thin blood or have a potent medical action, 1–2 cups is generally the standard limit and a therapeutic dose of these stronger herbs may be restricted to a set number of days to keep it all in safe proportions.

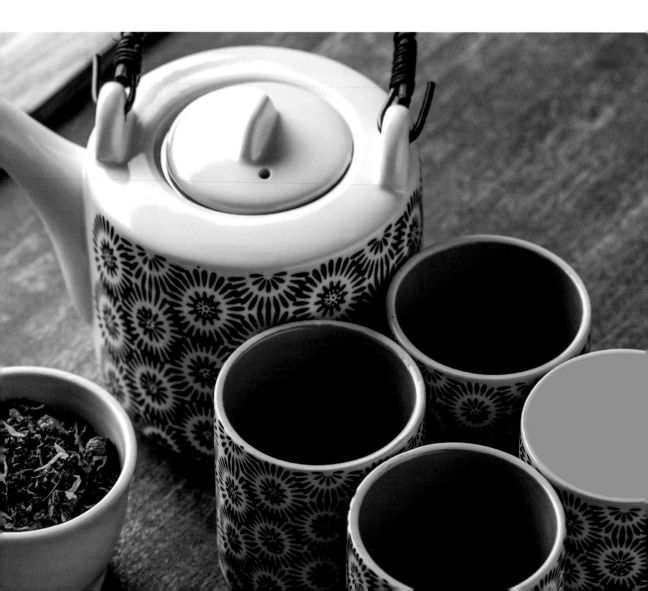

Some herbal teas are most effective in blocks with rest periods – that could be weekdays on, weekends off, or a week on, week off situation. In the dosage section within each entry, I give a rough guideline to dosage based upon the ratios listed and with consideration to the medicinal strength or actions of the herb. However, as an 'idealised' guide to dosage it cannot take into account your unique circumstances; for example, if you are taking the tea specifically for its decongestant action, you might limit the usage to the duration of the cold or allergy flare-up that you have. If you are taking it for another of its medicinal applications, however, that may warrant a several week or long-term usage.

Consultation with a herbalist will address correct dosage for your own physicality (age/height/weight) and medical history. So while there is a rough dosage guideline for each tea herb in this book, this is not an invitation to self-medicate without supervision; it is to show the current known safety parameters of the herb. Your constitution and personal medical history may make the guidelines invalid.

For some people opting to utilise herbal tea as a replacement to caffeine-containing beverages, consumption may rise to 4–5 cups, which is considered the upper limits of the milder teas. For example, this level of intake may take something like a sip of calming chamomile tea more into the realms of a drowsy, 'do not operate machinery' chamomile medication, as higher doses can intensify the action. Similarly, this level of consumption can also turn a gentle stimulant into a no sleep tonight affair. It's important to remember that these extra cups can bring on other medicinal actions beyond your intended use – for example, the subtle digestive support becomes a laxative.

So consideration to dosage (if using for therapeutic purposes) or attention to quantity (even just in the context of daily usage as a beverage) is an important matter. General guidance will be given within each individual entry.

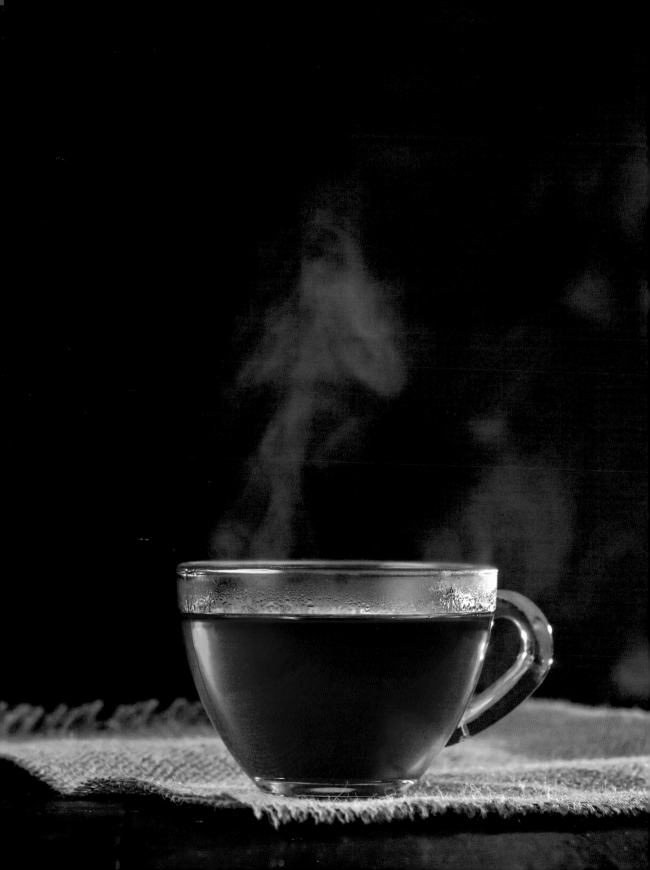

A Perfected Brew

Some herbal teas rely on their vitamin and mineral content to deliver their medicinal actions, while with others there are different phytochemicals at play. Some constituents are easily extracted via a short 1–4-minute infusion in boiling water as you would achieve while making a standard cup of tea. Others, however, require a longer steepage to fully extract their beneficial actions, or a temperature lower than boiling water to keep their volatile oils intact – chamomile for example. Volatile oils (aroma compounds or flavour molecules), as well as being plant chemicals, are often the essence of the taste experience. For other herbs – generally root-based or of woody parts – a different method altogether is required to effectively extract the health-supporting agents: a decoction or a pan simmering for up to 10–20 minutes.

Undercooking or overcooking can negate the benefit of the tea and its full flavour potential. So each entry indicates the best procedure to maximise both taste and benefit. This is not a book strictly about making medicine; it's about making a decent cup of tea that also has a decent bit of medicinal/healing action. Therefore, it is more a set of instructive recipe tips, so that we don't overcook the goodness or undervalue the strength of the ingredients.

Ratios

All my ratios are in relation to dried herbs – to mirror their equivalent in teabag form. Many of the herbs herein will come in loose tea or are easily sourced dried in a health store or food market. Fresh is often too short a season, whereas dried is year-round convenience.

My tea ratios are generally in the range of 1 teaspoon of chopped herbage per 1 cup of water.

Herbage	=	foliage, flower, crushed seed, root, berry and, in some instances, ground spice
1 teaspoon	=	approx. 4–5g of dried herb
1 cup	=	225–250ml (8 fl. oz)

This ratio delivers flavour and phytochemistry – i.e. the plant-based chemicals that activate our system towards healing or wellness – meaning there are good quantities of health constituents in each sip. The strength of the cup thus produced is average in scale to a cup of traditional herbal tea, as opposed to one of a strong medicinal extract. For example, thyme cough syrup as a strong medicinal extract would involve much more herbage in the mix and may involve other means of phytochemical extraction than hot water. Thyme tea, however, will be lightly expectorant (mucus clearing) and have the capacity to boost the immune system and fight the cough-causing bacteria or virus.

If you wish to strengthen the flavour – while making sure to take cautions and keep contraindications in mind, and ensuring that this is all okay with your system – then 2 teaspoons per cup is acceptable, rather than longer steepage, as longer steepage can extract more bitterness. Sometimes a long steepage can intensify phytochemical content but, on average, a standard infusion of 1–4 minutes will capture 50–90 per cent of the herb's phytochemistry and nutrients, and a similar quantity of flavour molecules.

The Rule of Thirds

This applies when substituting fresh for dried or vice versa. It's quite simple: 3 parts fresh herb = 1 part dried herb *OR* 1 unit of dry = 3 units fresh. Basically, this means that a teabag or a teaspoon of loose equates to 3 teaspoons of the freshly chopped herb.

The dried herb is more concentrated – when you think of it, the bulk of fresh is a high percentage of water, whereas the dried naturally has less water and volume but retains a considerable amount of its inherent phytoconstituents. So while it is more compact than fresh, it is still as full of healing properties.

Some dried herbs and spices will begin with a high percentage of phenols and antioxidants, but these can deteriorate over time. Storage away from light prolongs their shelf life. When it comes to fine powdered herbs and ground spices from the spice rack, they are more concentrated by volume than chopped, so the kitchen rule of thirds still applies and 1 teaspoon of standard crushed, dried herb can be substituted with a third of a teaspoon of powdered, dried herb.

Parts Used for Herbal Tea

The term 'herbal tea' applies to more than the herbaceous parts (foliage) of the plant; it can also apply to the seeds, roots and flowering parts. Your proprietary blend may not be a single constituent tea, but may have many plant parts or different parts from different herbs to enhance its flavour profile or medicinal actions. The following are types you may readily encounter.

Flowers/floral teas

Floral teas have a long history, the most common of which include chamomile, chrysanthemum, orange flowers, as well as hibiscus and jasmine, which are both herbal teas in their own right and flavour enhancers to tea blends. Whether fresh or dried, the flower buds, full blooms or picked petals may make up the infusion or flavour enhancement.

Foliage/leaf tea

The fresh or dried leaves of edible and often medicinal herbal plants make up the backbone of the catalogue of herbal teas.

Foliage plus

Sometimes foliage can be blended with other plant parts – so, for example, a proprietary brand of 'nettle tea' may be both dried root and dried foliage. Sometimes several plants and several parts may appear in a blend or mix – so, for example, lemon balm foliage may be mixed with chamomile flowers and valerian root to make a sleep or anti-anxiety tea.

Roots

The root systems of many plants contain their strongest concentration of phyto-chemicals and so are utilised in herbal teas and herbalism. This includes the likes of valerian, burdock, nettle and so on. Rarely are they used fresh, but are instead generally dried for storage and long-term use beyond a single season. Some may also be gently roasted before brewing, but I find that this can change the chicory root tea or nettle root into more of a coffee substitute than a tea.

Seeds

Several plants contain a microburst of nutrients, phytochemicals and a flavourful punch within their seeds, such as anise, fennel and star anise.

Fruit

Fresh fruits can be infused in hot water to yield a pleasing herbal tea, or in cold water to be served over ice as a refreshing beverage. Many fruits contain potent phytochemicals that make the tea remedial. Dried fruits can be utilised in a blend for flavour enhancement, or to avail of the medicinal principles of that plant.

Fruit Peels

Infusions from fresh or dried fruit peels, most popularly of citrus fruits, have a long history as flavour enrichers and aroma masks to strong medicinal plants, but they also contain medicinal chemistry. Lemon, orange and grapefruit are the most popular. Most of these are blended with the tea at production stage, but can also function as teas in their own right.

Other Factors

The Water Element

Lu Yu, author of *The Classics of Tea*, written in the eighth century, outlines the principles of brewing the perfect cup of tea, from the size of the water receptacle to the height from which water should be boiled above the fire. While this may seem a little complicated, one thing that still leaps out as being of supreme relevance today is the author's assertion that the best tea must be brewed with the best water.

The best water may be bottled spring water or filtered tap water, depending on your preference. The aim is to have a source of non-chlorinated water. Chlorine can affect the phytochemistry and taste of many herbs. A simple trick with tap water is to fill a pitcher and let it sit overnight, whereupon its ionic structure will alter and the chlorine will mostly dissipate.

Sourcing Herbal Tea

The herbal teas in this book are among the most popular teas consumed globally. They are pretty much all readily available in teabags from a variety of manufacturers on shelves in your local supermarket or health store. Quite a few are even to be found in convenience stores, corner shops and in the aisles at garden centres, gift shops and lifestyle stores. It really isn't that hard to find herbal teas.

The 'herbs' of the teas are also easily sourced in bulk or loose form. Dried herbage of foliage, flowers, seeds, bark strips and roots can be sourced year round from health stores and reputable online and mail-order suppliers. Growing your own is possible for many teas but not all – your local climate may not match the cultivation requirements of every plant on the list. But many are suitable to grow in your garden or in pots on a balcony; the culinary herbs, for example, will even thrive on a sunny windowsill. Apart from watering and caring, you will need to acquire more information on how to dry each herb for long-term storage, unless you intend to only utilise fresh and in-season herbs. There are many books on the subject and your local library or bookstore will ably assist you.

Storing Tea

Be it a teabag, loose tea or herbage (including seeds, bark, roots or dried fruits, etc.), proper storage is essential to ensure that your tea retains not just fragrance and flavour, but viability as a medicinal source. Tea/herbage can go off (structurally deteriorate, lose its constituents or even begin to decompose) over time, but this deterioration will accelerate if incorrect storage is allowed to happen.

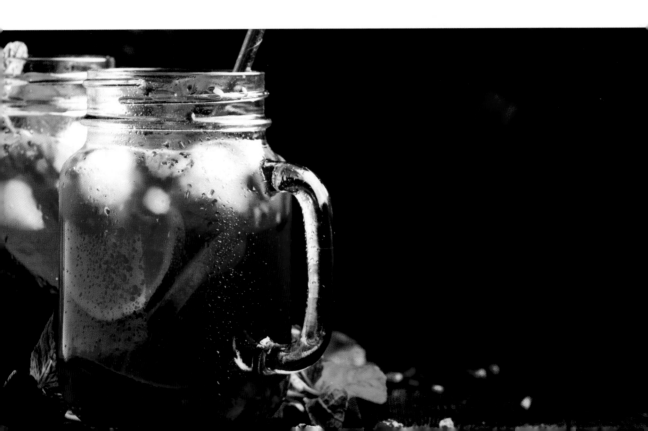

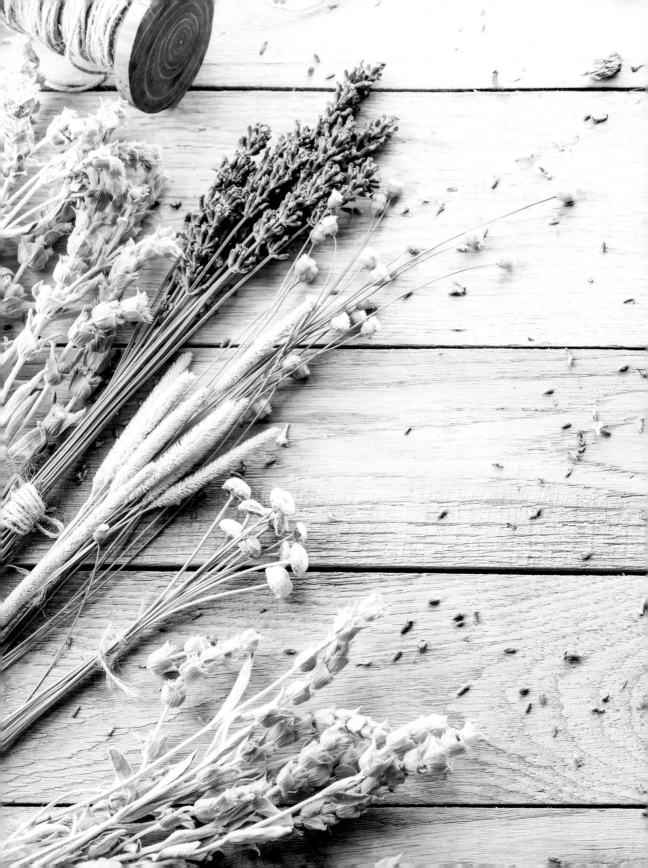

Container Types

Because tea can easily absorb moisture from the air and potentially begin to go mouldy, it is best kept in an airtight container. Traditional tea caddies are still available, but as people have varying preferences, other types of tins, containers, upcycled jam jars, kilner jars, etc., are all acceptable.

One note on glass is that prolonged light exposure will degrade tea, so, unless the glass is opaque, do make sure to store it in a dark cupboard. Glass jars can also be lined with greaseproof paper to lessen light entry. It's important to remember that glass can accelerate mould formation if moisture is allowed in.

Tea that comes in a foil packet can stay there, but it is a good tip to keep it sealed from excess air by employing a bulldog clip or elastic band, or decant it to a long-term storage container.

Porcelain/ceramic/earthenware containers are often porous to air and ambient moisture – especially if kept on a countertop or near the steam of a kettle – unless a tight lid and inner non-porous treatment are used. There are copper and tin caddies and modern tea-containers available to suit all types of herbage and tea types.

The only exception to all of the above is with pu-erh tea. With this, connoisseurs recommend that a degree of porousness in its tea caddy is required as its flavour improves over the course of its ageing process – hence the tradition of using porous Yixing tea storage pots.

Location

Tea and herbal tea should always be stored in a dry, cool, dark environment – traditionally inside the larder or kitchen cupboard, though, once upon a time it would have been placed in the tea chest or tea drawer. In the context of today, however, a shelf in your kitchen press will suffice. Although, as some people like to keep their herbs and teas handy and visible, I would note that some caddies sold as countertop storage require thought as to their placement – for example, make sure to pick a location that avoids temperature fluctuations and moisture absorption; also avoid exposure to kettle steam, cooking heat and direct sunlight, and close proximity to central heating.

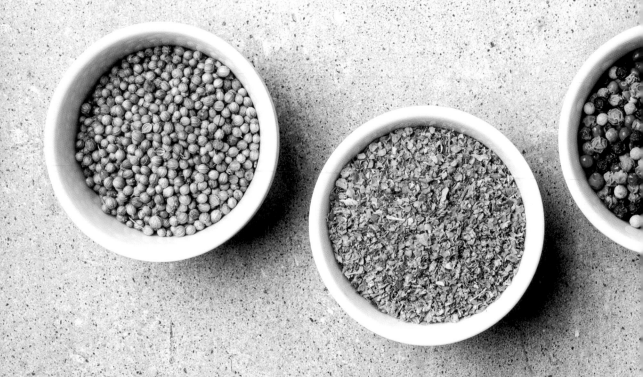

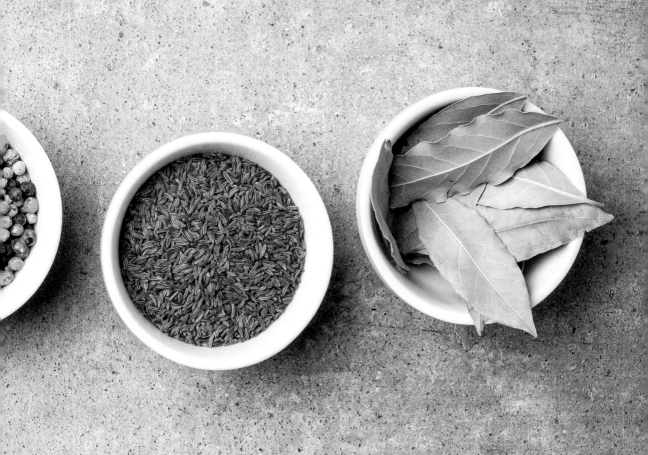

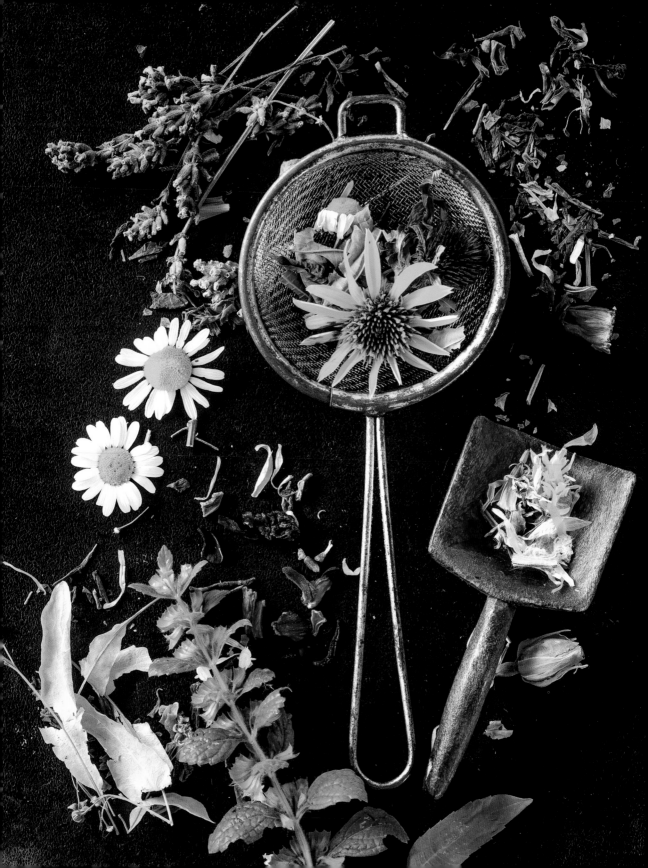

Making Tea

The Vessels

The Boiling Vessel

I won't go all Lu Yu on you, but I would recommend that you boil your water in something that is not aluminium lined, as the ions released under heat can interact with the phytochemicals and minerals of the plant. However, it can be aluminium on the outside with a ceramic inner. Likewise, many modern kettles are electric and plastic and, while regarded as safe, plastic does transfer some of its chemistry into boiling water. Therefore, copper pots and kettles come highly recommended.

The Brewing Vessel

I have a collection of teapots, but my favourite one is made of glass. I still get excited watching the water change colour as the herb surrenders its flavour and chemistry to the heat. It's like magic. And although I'm aware that it's just a psychological trick, seeing the process makes me believe in the healing properties of the tea even more. Any good teapot will do, but traits to look out for are a good pouring spout and a nice-fitting lid. As to volume capacity and colour, and matching it with your kitchen – well, that's all yours.

The Drinking Vessel

It's best if it's a glass, ceramic or china cup. Wooden or plastic cups can result in unwanted flavours (and in the case of plastics, undesirable chemistry, as previously explained) transferring into your hot water and adulterating your tea. And while any old mug will suffice, think of treating yourself to a special cup, one pleasing to the eye and nice to feel in your hand, as this maximises the pleasure experience of sipping herbal tea.

The Methods

Making a Standard Infusion

In herbalism, the terms 'tea' and 'infusion' are interchangeable – sometimes the word 'tisane' may be used. They are all basically the same thing – boiling or just off the boil water is added to a small portion of dried herb or fresh leaf or flower of a healing plant and allowed to infuse for generally between 3–7 minutes, then strained, after which the liquid can be drunk while either hot or cold. The ingredient ratios vary from remedy to remedy, but usually the average would be a teaspoon to a cup. More specific ratios will be given for each entry where required.

While the 3–7 minute rule can generally apply, some herbs may need shorter or longer exposure to heat than others, and so recommendations will be listed in each entry based on traditional practices. That said, there is new evidence around optimal steep time – be it in a cup or in a teapot. Apak (2006) recommends an infusion time of 5 minutes as the optimum for extracting antioxidants and polyphenols from true tea (*Camellia sinensis*). It was noted that if infused for longer than 5 minutes those compounds either precipitate or form floating clumps and so decrease in efficacy. So if you are making a herbal tea for its content of antioxidants and polyphenols, it is worth adhering to a 5-minute rule.

Teacup v Teapot

To make a pot of herbal tea

Place the herbage inside the teapot. Bring the kettle water to a boil and let it rest for 20–30 seconds to 1 minute, then pour it in over the herb. Place the lid on the pot and allow the liquid to steep for the required amount of time. If using loose herb, pour through a strainer and serve.

To make tea in a cup

Place the teabag or tea holder in the cup. Boil the kettle but allow the water to sit off the boil for a minimum of 20–30 seconds. Pour the hot water over the herbs once this period of time has elapsed. If you are using aromatic herbs where the medicine is in the volatile oils, or you simply want to maximise flavour, cover your cup with a saucer to prevent evaporation of the oils along with the steam. Allow the tea to steep for the required amount of time, remove the teabag/holder (and the saucer, if using) and serve.

A Strong Brew

Unlike with *Camellia sinensis* (black, green, white tea), where the stronger or longer you brew it, the more bitter it gets, herbal teas can be left to steep longer to let more phytochemical content leach out and yield a stronger dose of medicinal principles other than antioxidants and polyphenols. 'Brew', in this case, does not mean boiled for any particular length, as is the case with Senjiru or decoction methods (detailed below) – it is simply that the infusion/teabag can be allowed to sit for up to 10–20 minutes extra inside the cup or teapot and reheated if required. It can also be sipped cool. Moving from 1 teaspoon to 2 teaspoons will also deliver a stronger brew at the standard infusion duration.

Senjiru

A traditional Japanese method for brewing herbal teas that involves a rapid boiling of the plant part, followed by a 15-minute simmer and then a cool-down period of 10 minutes, before straining to serve the tea while it's still hot. Alternatively, it can be fully cooled and then chilled, or even served over ice. The ratio is generally 1 rounded tablespoon of herb to 2 cups of water.

Decoctions

Traditionally in herbalism a decoction is a sort of liquid soup, strained from the boiled or long-simmered parts of a healing plant. Sometimes several parts of a plant can be used (twigs, roots, berries, leaves and flowers) and up to several plants can appear in a decoction, depending on the remedy recipe.

Decoctions are generally cooked up in a saucepan or pot, or in a copper teapot. It is best to avoid aluminium pots/saucepans as the ions released under heat can interact with the phytochemical and mineral content of the plant.

When it comes to herbal teas, the boil or simmer method for a particularly long duration is often reserved for woody material or roots – the extra length of cooking is needed to fully extract the active agents from deeper inside these parts. The ingredient ratio of herb to liquid is usually 1oz to 1 pint or 25–30g to 500–600ml. The herb is placed in the water and simmered or boiled up to extraction temperatures.

The standard decoction method is to bring the parts to a boil, then simmer for 20 minutes, strain and allow the liquid to cool – only the strained liquid is used. Decoctions can often add some bitterness, so you can sweeten with honey or other options. Longer duration decoctions can apply to specific barks or roots. If required for any tea here it will be noted.

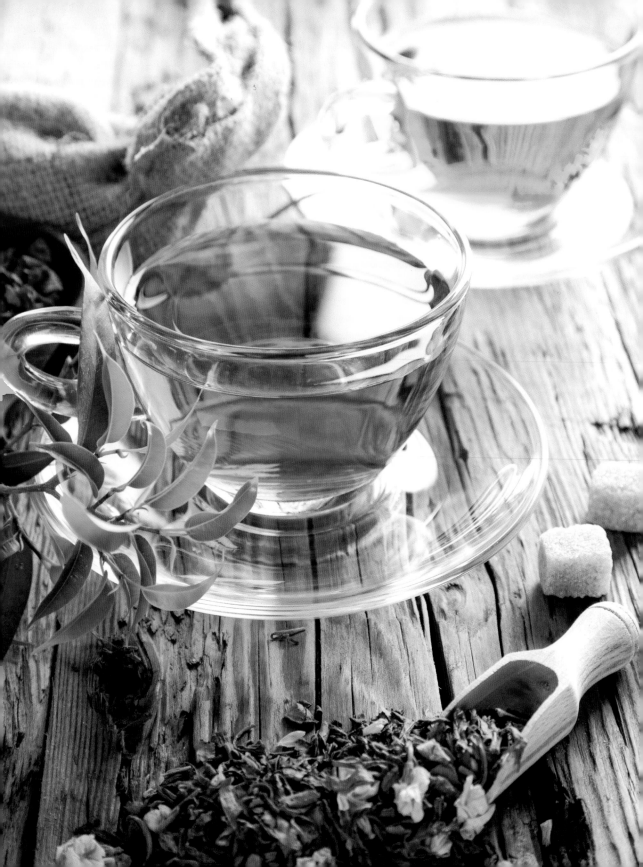

Some Other Options for Tea Making

'Sun tea' or a Sun Infusion

Often a method for floral essence teas or a ceremonial tea. Simply place the gently rinsed flower or the aromatic fresh/dried herb of choice into a glass or jar, fill with spring or filtered water and place into a window which catches the sun. Allow this liquid to steep and infuse for several hours, then make sure to remove any solids from the infusion before serving. Once ready, the liquid can be chilled or served over ice.

'Moon tea' or a Lunar Infusion

Similar to sun tea but the infusion period is instead carried out overnight in a window that catches the moonlight. Drink first thing in the morning. Can also be chilled or served over ice.

Iced Tea

Make your herbal tea by any method above. Cool fully and refrigerate to serve chilled over ice.

Some Notes on Sweeteners and Additives

Milk and Sugar?

As a rule, herbal tea is generally not diluted with milk (even nut or soya substitutes). Cow's milk is viewed as an adulterant that not only alters flavour but may actually alter the properties of the herb or the uptake of its phytochemicals. Furthermore, herbal teas with high tannins and other phytoconstituents can curdle milk and so just ruin the cup. Sugar is also seen as an adulterant and can impact on both the efficacy and true flavour of the herbal tea.

Artificial Sweeteners

In some quarters these are a health revolution and in others are considered to be excitotoxins (chemicals that are disruptive to the nervous and endocrine systems). More research needs to be carried out on dosage, duration of use, etc. The two most utilised are aspartame and saccharin.

Aspartame

Much lauded as having zero calories for all its sweet taste (some brands are said to be up to 200 times sweeter than that of sucrose/sugar), but the compound breaks down in the human system into phenylalanine, which inhibits the activity of a gut enzyme called alkaline phosphatase (ALP) known to slow the progression of metabolic syndrome, obesity and diabetes.

Saccharin aka sodium saccharin (benzoic sulfimide)

A manufactured sweetener approximately 300–400 times as sweet as sucrose/sugar (some brands claim to be up to 700 times as sweet). It can, however, have a bitter or metallic aftertaste. It will raise glucose levels, but not as strikingly as sugar. It belongs to a class of compounds known as sulfonamides, which can cause allergic reactions in some.

'Natural' Sweeteners

There are increasing numbers of natural choices on health store and supermarket shelves. Here are some of the more popular ones.

Agave syrup (extracted from Agave tequilana)

Sweeter than honey and table sugar but with a low glycaemic index, this is often promoted as a healthy alternative for diabetics. It is predominantly made up of fructans and fructose rather than glucose, and so absorbs more steadily and slowly into the bloodstream. Caveat – fructose is calorie high and while theoretically less damaging than table sugar it is no 'health compound' and can contribute to raised triglycerides and fat accumulation. The syrup, however, does contain quantities of iron, magnesium, calcium and potassium.

Erythritol

A derivative of plant-based sugar alcohol (occurring naturally in some fruit and fermented foods) that is processed into a low-calorie sweetener. It is roughly 60–80 per cent as sweet as sucrose (table sugar), but it does not spike blood glucose or insulin levels and has no impact upon cholesterol or triglycerides either. Overuse can cause some digestive upset.

Honey

This is so sweet because it consists almost completely of pure glucose and levulose (a fructose) and it will spike blood glucose and insulin. This is often overlooked, however, as it has so many other health benefits, which is mainly due to its mineral-rich and organic acid profile that supports liver function and intestinal health. Darker-coloured honey is higher in mineral and acid content.

Maple Syrup (extract of the sap of Acer saccharum)

Sweet by virtue of being approximately two-thirds sucrose, and with that comes all the links to obesity, type 2 diabetes and heart disease. It is seen as a healthier option in that, as a replacement option, gram for gram, it technically cuts sugar consumption by one-third and also because it is slower to trigger a spike. Maple syrup is a good source of manganese and zinc and can potentially yield around 20–30 different antioxidants, the darker ones more so.

Stevia (an extract from the leaves of Stevia rebaudiana)

This comprises two particularly sweet compounds – stevioside and rebaudioside A – each being around 100 times sweeter than sugar, gram for gram. It has zero calories and a zero rating on the glycaemic load index. In fact, it has been shown to improve insulin sensitivity and to reduce oxidised LDL cholesterol. Before its use as a sweetener, the herb had a medicinal value in reducing arterial plaque build-up.

Xylitol

A plant-based sugar alcohol. Traditionally found in birch trees, it can also be found in other sources that contain the plant fibre xylan. Its sweetness is on a par with sugar but with two-thirds of the calorific value. Xylitol does not spike blood sugar or insulin levels, and some scientific studies have shown that it can even improve bone density and so lower the risk of osteoporosis. It is fast becoming a replacement in dental-care products, as it supports remineralisation of teeth.

Yacon Syrup

New 'healthy syrups' come on the market all the time, but Yacon syrup looks promising as a natural sweetener. Beyond its potential to regulate blood sugar and cholesterol levels, it is quite high in fructooligosaccharides – a set of soluble fibres which feed and nurture bifidobacteria and lactobacilli (the good bacteria) in the intestines. It can, however, exert laxative properties in large doses.

Flavour Enhancers

Teas can be flavoured with all sorts of spices, other herbs and fruit juices or fruit slices. Here are the four most traditional:

Lemon juice/slice (Citrus Limonum)

Rich in vitamin C and limonin glucosides. Limonin is a potent anticarcinogen that also exhibits a cholesterol-lowering effect. Lemon juice is beneficial to stimulating our body's natural detoxifying processes. The aroma of a slice or splash within tea is stimulating and known to improve concentration, mood and energy perception, while decreasing anxiety, stress, nervousness and tension.

Lime juice/slice (Citrus aurantifolia)

Not only a source of antioxidant and immune-enhancing vitamin C, lime also contains limonoids, which have been shown to help inhibit cancers of the mouth, lung, breast, skin, stomach and colon. Lime juice may enhance iron absorption and so be useful to remedy anaemia (yet unhelpful to haemochromatosis – high iron in blood). It may – in doses higher than those used to sweeten tea – also slow or accelerate the activity of other minerals and phytochemicals.

Vanilla pod/extract (the extract/seed pods of Vanilla planifolia)

One of the most popular flavours globally. Its taste and aroma is considered to exert a calming influence, but perhaps its success is down to its ability to increase levels of catecholamines (including dopamine, norepinephrine and adrenaline), which trigger a slight addictive hit. It is anti-inflammatory and antioxidant in nature.

Cinnamon spice

Not just a feature of spiced cha, it is often utilised to 'sweeten' a bitter or bland tea, or indeed as a deliberate dose of medicinal spice – as a carminative and antispasmodic (to settle stomach and prevent spasms). Studies have shown that half a teaspoon daily can, over a couple of weeks, begin to lower cholesterol and triglyceride levels by as much as 20 per cent and help regulate blood sugar in non-insulin-dependent type 2 diabetes.

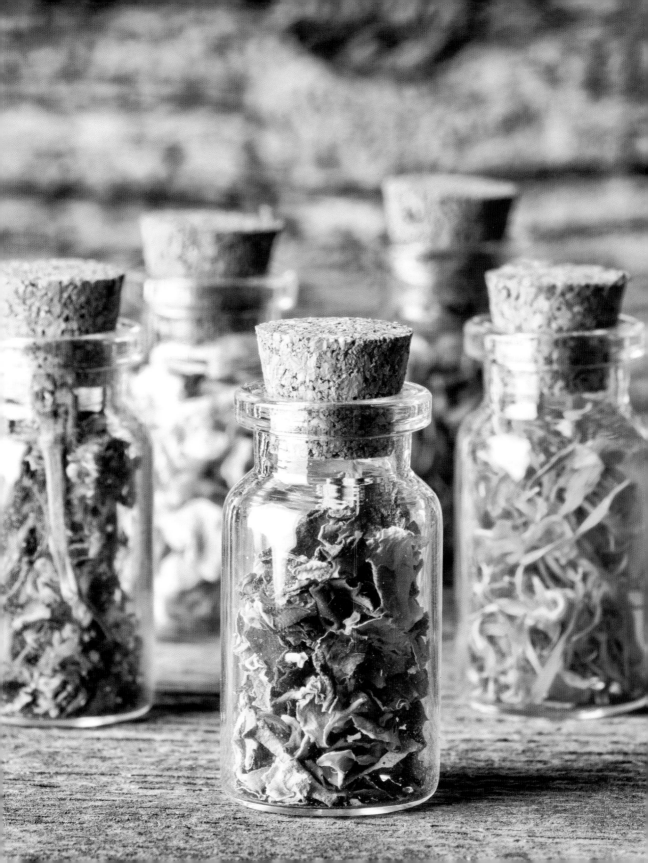

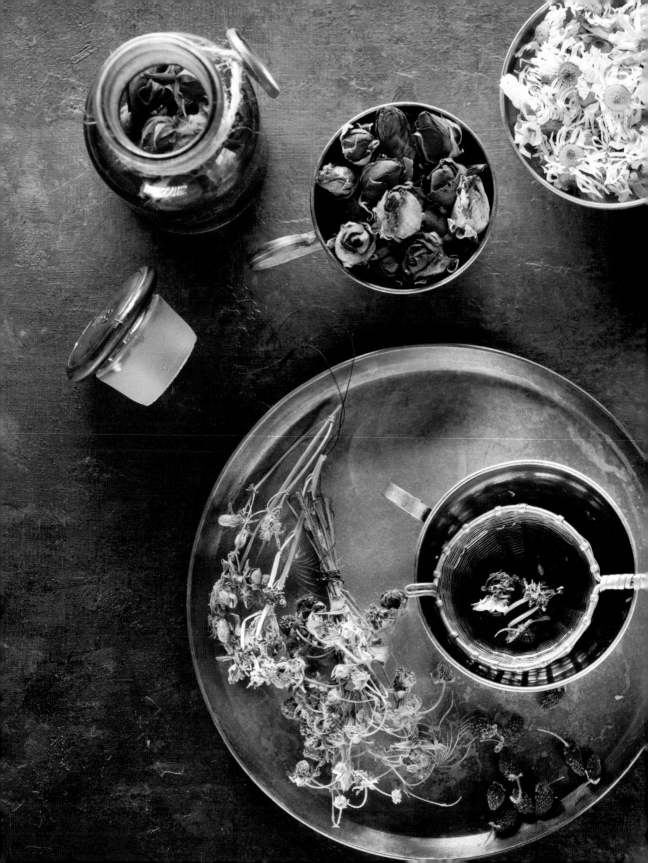

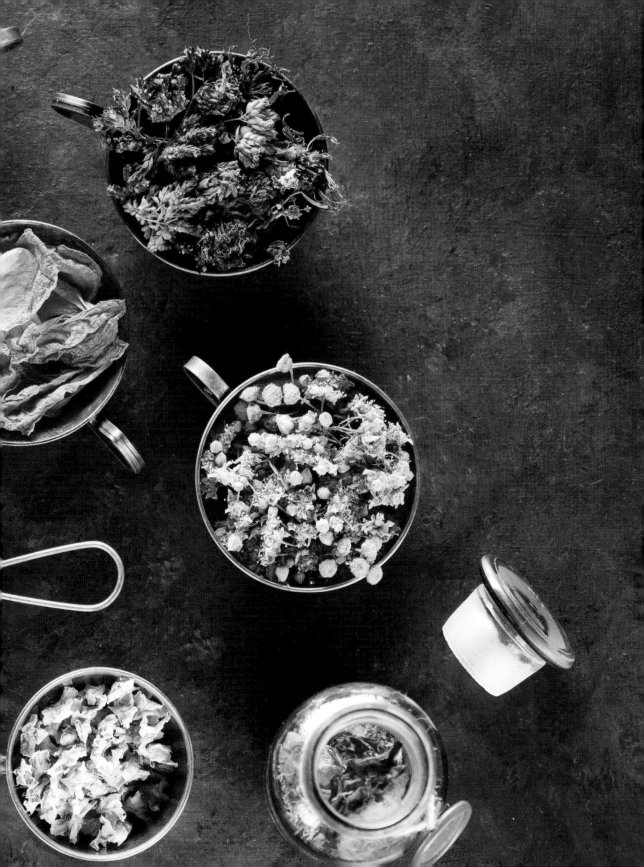

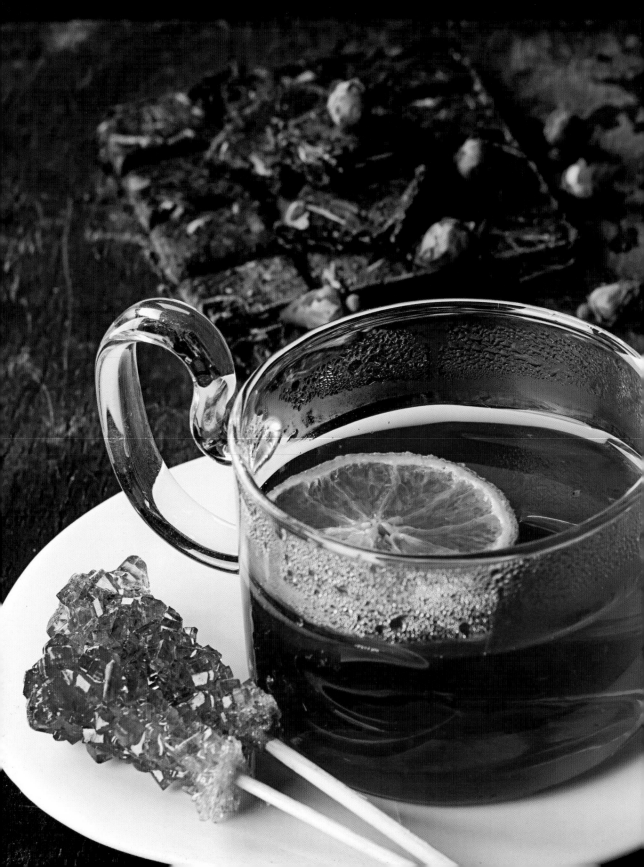

Directory of Herbal Teas

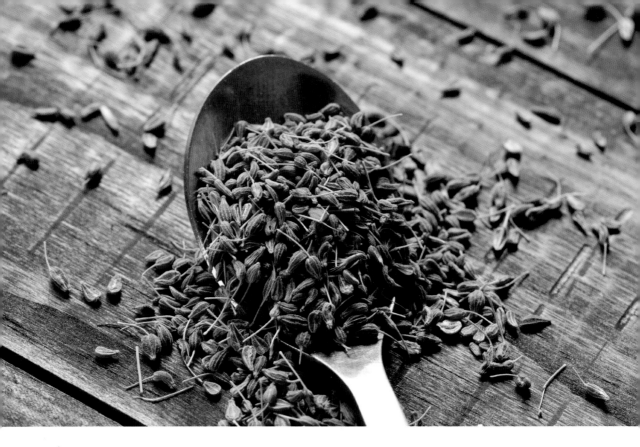

Anise Tea

(Pimpinella anisum)

Botanical family
Apiaceae/Umbelliferae

Parts used
Leaves and/or seeds

Flavour profile
Liquorice-like

Anise is one of the oldest known and still most popular spices. Cultivated globally, it was initially indigenous to the Mediterranean and the Nile delta, where it has been part of the agriculture and ethno-medicine of those regions for over 4,000 years. Its distinctive flavour is often employed to sweeten other herbal tea brews and commercial blends.

How to make

A tea can be made from leaf or seed. The leaf, however, is not as enriched as the seed. As it is the flavour molecules and the volatile oils that make this tea special, it is best to make an infusion with hot water that has boiled but been rested for 30–60 seconds before pouring. It is also essential to cover the cup or put the lid on the pot after pouring in the hot water in order to prevent heavy evaporation of those molecules.

Allow the tea to infuse for 2–4 minutes. Ratios (fresh or dried) of leaf or seed are generally kept to 1 teaspoon per cup of water or ⅓ teaspoon of ground spice. Anise tea is also available in teabags.

Health benefits

Mentioned in Pharaonic medical texts as a digestive and pain-relieving, anise spice and tea has a long history in remedial application. In contemporary herbalism its expectorant and antispasmodic actions see it utilised for respiratory and bronchial complaints – from cough to asthma and bronchitis. Being antimicrobial, it is often employed as a gargle against infections of the mouth and this, combined with its diuretic nature, means it is drunk to address urinary tract infections.

Anise can increase iron absorption, which is useful in remedying acute anaemia. It has a long history as a natural antacid to combat heartburn and is utilised to quell gastric upset and stomach pains, as well as helping improve digestion and alleviate bloating/flatulence. It is sometimes availed of for its oestrogenic action – the seeds in particular contain trans-anethole, a plant hormone very similar to human oestrogen, and therefore has traditionally been utilised to promote the onset of delayed or irregular menstruation, and as a support to lactation in nursing mothers.

Main medicinal actions: Analgesic, antibacterial, antimicrobial, antiseptic, antispasmodic, appetite stimulant, carminative, diaphoretic, digestive, diuretic, expectorant, galactagogue, oestrogenic, pancreatic stimulant, stomachic.

Dosage

Being potent, the traditional recommendation is to not exceed 2–3 cups per day, although a single cup will suffice as a dose. This can be refrigerated and sipped a little at each meal time.

Caution

The strong oestrogen-like action is best avoided during pregnancy and if suffering from endometriosis and oestrogen-reactive cancers. Use cautiously if you have issues with epilepsy, diabetes and blood pressure.

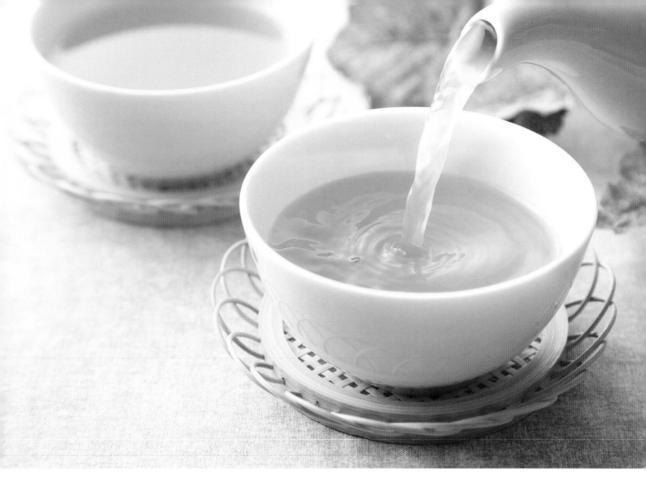

Artichoke Tea

(Cynara cardunculus var. scolymus)

Botanical family
Asteraceae

Parts used
Leaves and/or immature flower buds

Flavour profile
Sweet, vegetal

Artichoke is an herbaceous perennial in the thistle family, traditionally cultivated as a vegetable. Artichoke tea mainly refers to a tea of the foliage, although a popular Vietnamese tea known as atiso tea utilises the flower heads, and some blends mix both parts.

How to make
Artichoke leaf tea and atiso tea are both available in teabag form and so a standard infusion of 2–7 minutes will yield all its goodness and full flavour. You can make from fresh leaf or dried herb with a similar length infusion time. Artichoke leaf tea can have a slight grassy or vegetal flavour, which can translate as subtle sweetness.

Because of its culinary connection, some sources recommend a decoction method – boiling the leaf for some minutes, generally in the range of 5–10 – but there is no need to cook it up every time. Instead, you can simply finely chop a segment of leaf and add 1 teaspoon of it per cup of water. Boiling water is acceptable, but utilising just-off-the-boil water will keep some of the herb's antioxidant phenols more intact and extend its healthy offerings.

Health benefits

Artichoke leaf tea is recognised as a bitter tonic, containing higher concentrations of the phytochemical cynarin than the immature flower head. Cynarin and other bitter principles stimulate the liver and gall bladder to increase the production of bile and digestive enzymes that break down ingested fats and toxic accumulations of waste within the body. This process not only improves digestion and helps with the alleviation of bloating, belching, flatulence and heartburn, etc., but by prompting natural detoxification and combining the plant's diuretic potential, it is remedial to arthritis, gout, inefficient kidney function and liver disease. Cynarin and artichoke's other major component, silymarin, can help to support regeneration of liver cells and both also contribute to lower blood glucose, serum cholesterol and triglyceride levels. Artichoke tea is gaining respect as an adjunct treatment to irritable bowel syndrome (IBS).

Main medicinal actions: Antibacterial, antidyspeptic, antihyperlipidaemic, anti-inflammatory, cholagogue, detox, diabetic control, diuretic, weight loss.

Dosage

As a pleasant tea there is no particular guide limit, but in general the remedial recommendation is to have a cup around half an hour before each meal for a week or so until the problem resolves, or a cup before a particularly fatty or stodgy meal.

Caution

Avoid if allergic to ragweed or other members of the Asteraceae family. Use under supervision with liver, kidney or gall bladder disease and also with gallstones.

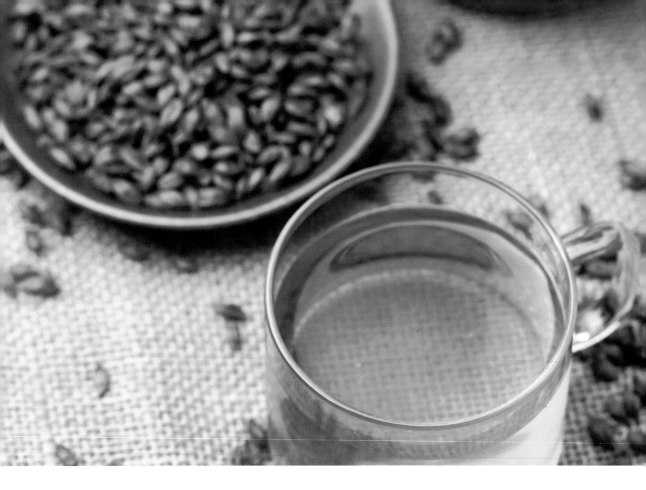

Barley Tea

(Hordeum vulgare)

Botanical family

Gramineae

Parts used

Grain

Flavour profile

Roasted, bitter

Barley is a cereal grain with a rich nut-like flavour. It has a history of use and cultivation dating back to the first non-nomadic civilisations. Roasted barley grain infusions are popular across Japan, Korea and China. In Japan, barley tea is known as *mugi-cha*; in Korea, as *bori-cha*, while in China, barley tea may be called *dàmài-chá* or *mài-chá*.

How to make

The toasted/roasted grain attains a rich flavour with slightly bitter undertones. Barley can be roasted at home in the oven or a hot pan, or found ready roasted in Asian markets and some health stores. Powdered dried barley may also be found.

1–2 teaspoons of roasted, unhulled barley kernels per cup is required. Traditionally brewed via the Senjiru method for anywhere from 5 to 15 minutes, longer brews have a more intense flavour and may veer into the category of 'coffee substitute'. A 2–5-minute infusion is also possible. The tea, however you make it, can be served hot, cold or over ice.

Health benefits

Barley tea is known as a night-time beverage that supplies a restful sleep and certainly it supplies a source of both tryptophan and mela-tonin – both of which trigger brain chemistry responses that promote relaxed states, sleepiness and deeper, more restorative sleep. It has a good reputation for promoting appetite and assisting with efficient digestion – but unlike most acidity-raising digestives, it is a natural ant-acid, availed of to help prevent acid reflux and utilised as a soothing tonic to the stomach in recovery from gastric upset or viral infection.

Considered a detox beverage because it prompts urination and toxic clearance, and also promotes healthy bowel movements, barley also supplies insoluble fibre that feeds probiotic and other friendly bacteria in the intestinal tract. It is a source of beta-glucans, which actively slow the absorption of glucose and help to reduce total cholesterol, LDL and triglycerides. It has the potential to delay or protect the system from atherosclerosis, diabetes, cardiovascular disease and stroke.

Furthermore, barley contains hordenine – a phenethylamine alkaloid that alleviates bronchial spasms and chest tightness and may be useful with asthma and seasonal allergy. Hordenine also boosts both metabolism and physical endurance.

Main medicinal actions: Antacid, anti-diabetic, antioxidant, anti-cholesterol, circulatory tonic, detox, digestive, diuretic, hypnotic, laxa-tive, stomachic, restorative, venotonic, weight loss.

Dosage

1–2 cups per day will provide the therapeutic trick.

Caution

Avoid if coeliac or if you have an intolerance to gluten grains. May increase the effectiveness of diabetic and anticoagulant medication.

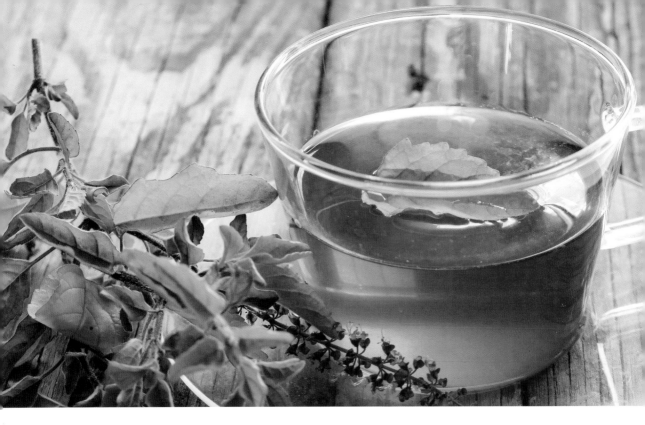

Basil, Holy, aka Tulsi Tea

(Ocimum sanctum syn. Ocimum tenuiflorum)

Botanical family
Lamiaceae

Parts used
Leaves

Flavour profile
Sweet, peppery

Holy Basil, aka tulsi, has been cultivated as a culinary herb and medicinal plant in India for more than 5,000 years. And while it is popularly known as a traditional libido enhancer and contraceptive/antifertility agent in Ayurvedic medicine, it has much wider health applications.

How to make
Tulsi tea is readily available in teabag form and suits a standard infusion at 3–7 minutes steepage time. Because lots of the healing agents are in the volatile oils and so easily evaporate, I like to brew it in a teapot, or cover the cup with a saucer for the duration of the steepage.

If utilising fresh leaf, then shredding or tearing the leaf allows for more phytochemicals to leach into your hot water, which is best delivered to the herb around 30 seconds after boiling. Fresh leaf phytochemicals can evaporate more quickly than dried. The ratio – be it dry or fresh – is generally 1 teaspoon per cup of water – but note that dry herb is often stronger flavoured. In all forms it offers an intensive, sweet-camphorous flavour and aroma.

Health benefits

The antifertility reputation is backed up by studies, indicating that regular use can lower sperm count levels in males and diminish luteinising hormones and follicle-stimulating hormones in females. The libido enhancing for both male and female may be down to a combination of circulation boosting and general well-being enhancement after the antioxidant and adaptogenic (stress stabilising) actions take effect.

Beyond the bedchamber of the gods, tulsi has traditionally had a role in respiratory support and in the treatment of bronchial ailments, including asthma. It has decongestant, expectorant and antitussive (lessens cough reflex) properties that have seen it employed with relief to colds and flus too. Its nutrient and phytochemical array (including apigenin, beta-sitosterol, eugenol, rosmarinic acid, myretenal and luteolin) have seen modern herbalists utilise it for adrenal fatigue, hypothyroidism, depression, anxiety, metabolic syndrome and obesity.

Tulsi tea also has a role in detoxification via its antioxidant, diaphoretic and diuretic activity. It is a good source of dietary ursolic acid, which is a selective COX-2 inhibitor – so delivering both anti-inflammatory and some cancer-preventing activity. It also has applications in improving cognitive function and inhibiting dementia decline.

Main medicinal actions: Adaptogen, antibacterial, antifertility, anti-hyperglycaemic, antioxidant, antitussive, carminative, decongestant, detox, diaphoretic, diuretic, expectorant, immunomodulatory, stomachic, neuroprotective.

Dosage

Therapeutic dosage is in the range of 1 to a maximum of 3 cups daily.

Caution

Can increase the effect of blood-thinning medication and affect natural coagulation. May impact upon glucose levels and diabetic medications.

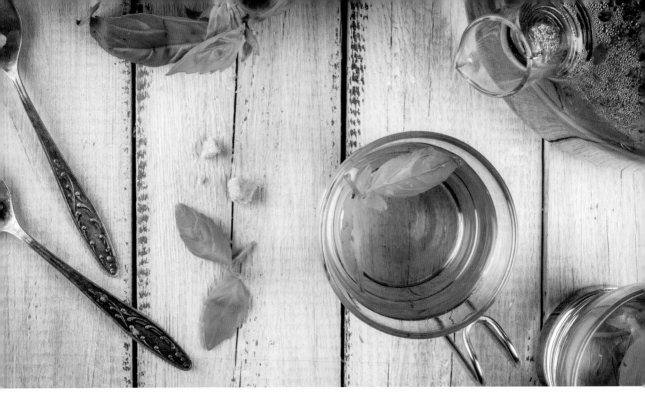

Basil, Sweet, Tea

(*Ocimum basilicum*)

Botanical family
Lamiaceae

Parts used
Leaves

Flavour profile
Sweet, peppery

Ocimum basilicum, also known as sweet basil, is an annual plant from the mint family with a long history as a culinary herb. The genus name *Ocimum* derives from the ancient Greek word *ozo*, meaning 'to smell', and certainly basil emits a pleasant aroma. There are several cultivars of basil, including lemon and cinnamon-scented varieties, as well as the foliage shape variations such as Italian/curly basil and lettuce leaf basil.

How to make

Sweet basil is best served by a standard infusion of 3–5 minutes duration. Ensure you cover it in order to trap all the flavour molecules and health-supporting volatile oils. The ratio is generally 1–2 teaspoons of shredded foliage (shredding helps release more of its constituents than an intact leaf) per cup of boiling water. Sweet basil tea, as its name suggests, is on the sweeter side and is less pungent/bitter than other varieties of basil. It has a subtle peppery tang, but if infused for too long it becomes increasingly bitter. Also makes a wonderful iced tea.

Health benefits

Basil tea is a traditional treatment for anaemia and fatigue. It is a good source of iron to build healthy haemoglobin and thus also improve the oxygen-carrying capacity of the blood. As a bitter tonic, it has agency with stimulating liver function and so is often engaged as a detox or cleanse tea. The tea is useful in boosting digestion and has a role in alleviating bloating and trapped wind. It also can address gastritis and other stomach ailments.

Sweet basil tea contains many polyphenolic flavonoids with potent antioxidant value and so is seen as a healthy beverage. Many of its polyphenolic compounds have been shown to exhibit significant anti-inflammatory activity. Eugenol, for example, inhibits the inflammatory cyclooxygenase enzymes (COX 1 and 2) responsible for flare-ups of rheumatoid arthritis, osteoarthritis and inflammatory bowel conditions, and which can contribute to the progression of atherosclerosis, and neurodegenerative and cardiovascular diseases.

Sweet basil is a source of myrcene and linalool – two primary terpenes shared with hops, cannabis and other sedative and pain-relieving plants. The tea taken by day has a tradition in mild pain management and injury recovery, while at night its consumption has tradition as a relaxant and sleep promoter.

Main medicinal actions: Adaptogen, analgesic, anti-anxiety, anti-bacterial, antihyperglycaemic, anti-inflammatory, antimutagenic, anti-oxidant, antispasmodic, antitussive, carminative, decongestant, detox, diaphoretic, digestive, diuretic, expectorant, immunomodulatory, neuroprotective, sedative, stomachic.

Dosage

Generally kept within the range of 2–3 cups a day.

Caution

Sweet basil can augment the efficacy of insulin and blood glucose-lowering medications, so caution/guidance in taking this is required with all diabetes types (including gestational).

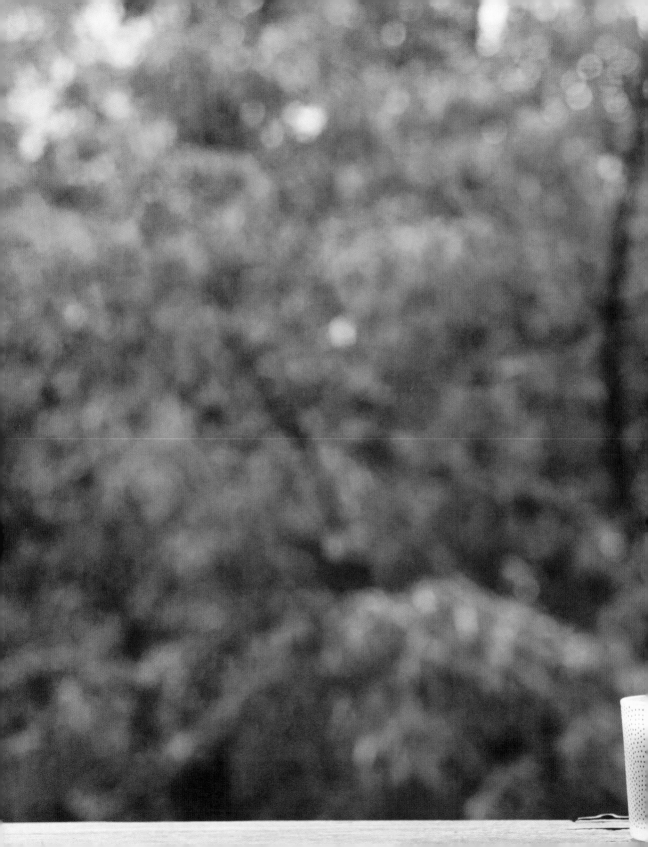

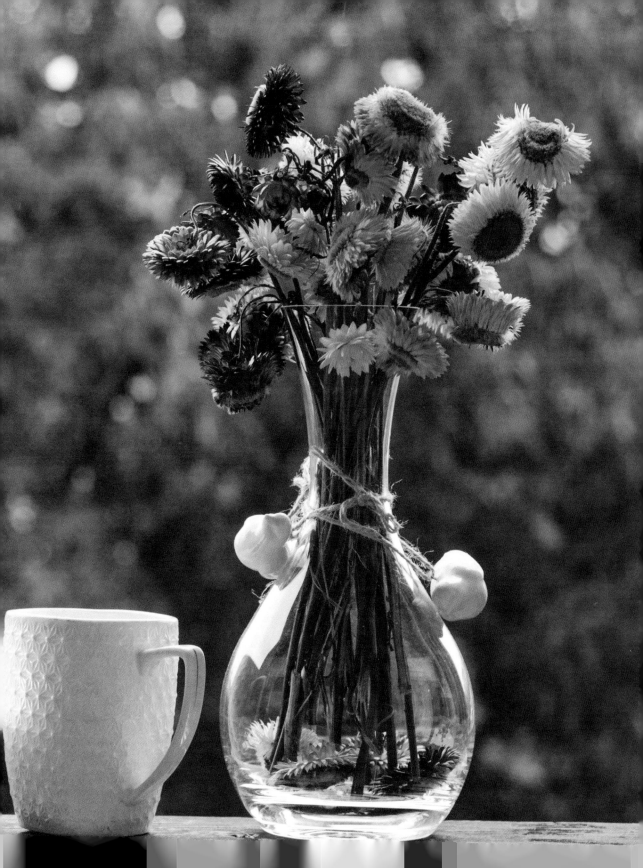

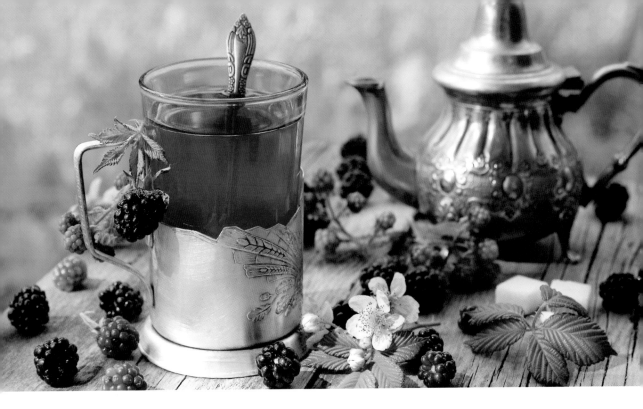

Blackberry Fruit Tea

(*Rubus fruticosus*)

Botanical family
Rosaceae

Parts used
Fruit

Flavour profile
Tangy, sweet

While blackberry foliage has been the medicinal tea of choice throughout the history of herbalism, with the fruits reserved for nutrition and dietary medicine, in recent years blackberry fruit teas and blackberry-flavoured green or white teas have found a place in the canon of herbal health teas. The nutrients, soluble fibre, fruit acids and phytochemicals that leach from the fruit into the hot water deliver some rewarding benefits when imbibed.

How to make

Blackberry fruit tea can be made from a teaspoon or two of dried or fresh berries infused in boiling water which has rested a moment – allow to soak for a duration of 3–7 minutes before straining the berries away. There are commercial brands of blackberry tea that may contain other fruits and herbs in the blend – the infusion rate here is the same but the flavour and medicinal profile will reflect the additional ingredients. Blackberry tea is also pleasant as an iced tea.

Health benefits

Blackberries are particularly loaded with vitamin C, which sees the beverage often availed of to fight against seasonal illness and in recuperation. But it is important to keep in mind that vitamin C is also a scavenger of pro-inflammatory molecules and of compromised oxygen molecules known as free radicals, which damage blood vessels and cause cellular deterioration. The richness of blackberry's anthocyanins further benefits venous health and quells inflammations. The fruit's content of manganese is a further combatant against inflammation.

The impressive levels of phenolic flavonoids, including quercetin, cyanidin and ellagic acid, show its antihistamine promise and also its protective actions against the progression of neurological diseases. The fruit contains pelargonidins, which protect what are known as endothelial cells – these line the interior surface of both blood vessels and lymphatic vessels, and maintain circulatory health. Pelargonidins help increase insulin sensitivity, while its catechin content also improves vascular function and brings about a better metabolism of glucose.

Blackberries are packed with phenolics, polyphenols and flavonoids, each exerting antioxidant and anti-inflammatory actions beneficial to arthritis, gout, psoriasis, etc. Many of those same phytochemicals also have antiviral and antiproliferative (inhibits tumour cell growth) actions. The fruits also have a long standing as being chemopreventive – with their content of cyanidin 3-glucoside and ellagic acid supporting that cancer-protective potential.

Main medicinal actions: Anti-diabetic, antihistamine, anti-inflammatory, antioxidant, antiproliferative, antiviral, chemopreventive, convalescence support, diuretic, immune support.

Dosage

Generally within the range of 1–3 cups daily. The fruits have high fructose levels, which limits their therapeutic potential if overindulged.

Caution

Avoid if allergic to salicylic acid (aspirin), and it may also increase the potency of anticoagulant medication.

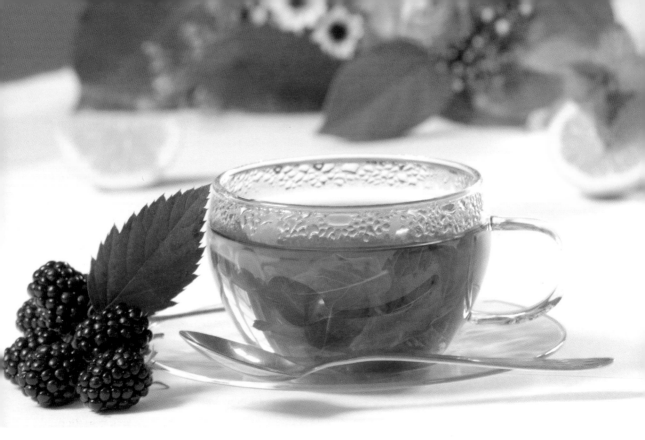

Blackberry Leaf Tea

(Rubus fruticosus)

Botanical family
Rosaceae

Parts used
Leaves

Flavour profile
Tannin to tart-sweet

Around the globe there is a range of approximately 2,000 microspecies of this woody-stemmed, thorny, fruit-bearing plant from the rose family. The plant that supplies our herbal tea is sometimes referred to as 'European blackberry' in order to distinguish it from other closely related North American and Australian *Rubus* species with less medicinal value.

How to make
Traditionally made from the dried leaves, which are infused for 5–10 minutes at a ratio of 1–2 teaspoons per cup of boiling water. Fresh foliage in a similar portion is also amenable to a standard infusion of 3–7 minutes. The flavour of the pure leaf tea is slightly bitter, but it can be sweetened with honey or other sweeteners to improve the taste.

Some proprietary blackberry blends may also include root and/or fruit extract and this can change the flavour to sweet-tart or closer to the fruit flavour of blackberry, depending on the ratio of parts. Dried or fresh fruit can be added at the beginning of the infusion or for the last 2 minutes of steepage, to enhance flavour and to add some extra vitamin C and beneficial antioxidants.

Health benefits

The Roman legions 2000-plus years ago were prescribed blackberry foliage to treat wounds and alleviate fatigue. Certainly topical applications of the tannin-rich tea has a function in cleaning and tightening cuts and also in improving common skin complaints from pimples to rashes. The foliage contains vitamin C, which promotes tissue repair topically, and which strengthens the immune system and metabolism when taken internally.

The foliage also contains anti-inflammatory and antiviral agents, such as flavonoids, saponins, glycosides, terpenoids and sterols. Blackberry leaf tea can help to inhibit the activity of interleukin-1 alpha – a protein directly linked to the production of inflammation molecules and which is associated with fever, sepsis, rheumatoid arthritis and gout, irritable bowel and digestive upset, tinnitus, diabetic neuropathy, pain hypersensitivity, lupus, endometriosis and Alzheimer's.

Globally, the tea is further utilised as an astringent tea to remedy diarrhoea and to calm mouth/throat inflammations. Some blends of blackberry tea can include the roots, which have a history of use in remedies for breaking up bladder stones and promoting urination.

Main medicinal actions: Anti-diabetic, antidiarrhoeal, anti-inflammatory, antiviral, astringent, decongestant, detox, diuretic, immune support, uterine stimulant.

Dosage

Best within the limits of 1–3 cups daily.

Caution

While considered antidiarrhoeal, overuse can exert a laxative effect. Blackberry leaves also share many phytochemicals with raspberry leaf, a noted uterine tonic: see p. 172.

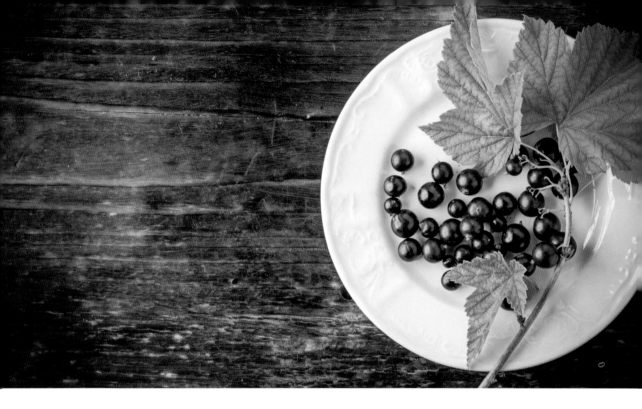

Blackcurrant Tea

(Ribes nigrum)

Botanical family
Grossulariaceae

Parts used
Leaves and berries

Flavour profile
Tannin to fruity

Blackcurrants often enter the 'superfood' charts with their potent anti-oxidant value and plenty of good nutrition, but the tea also has a long history in herbal health. Generally it consists of a mix of dried leaf and dried berry, but it can come as pure leaf alone, both loose and in tea-bags. Some blended brands may include black or green tea leaves or other herbs. Garden-sourced teas can utilise fresh foliage and berries.

How to make

Best by infusion at a duration of 1–3 minutes for a soft flavour and 3–7 minutes for a deeper brew. Standard ratio of 1 teaspoon per cup of water. To better avail of the vitamin C content, which can disintegrate at higher temperatures, use hot water that has rested off the boil for 40–60 seconds.

Shred fresh leaves for best effect. Depending on your blend (quantity of fruit in the mix), the tea will yield a pleasant aroma with a subtly sweet or tangy flavour. Pure leaf has a tannin-rich quality somewhat similar to a mild black tea. To make a purely fruit tea you can use 1 teaspoon of dried fruits per cup of hot water, or 3–4 fresh fruits (sliced or crushed). Strain the solids after a 4-minute infusion. Also suitable chilled and served over ice.

Health benefits

Both blackcurrant fruits and foliage contain not just vitamin C but flavonols, phenolic acids and esters, anthocyanins and procyanidins, all of which exert strong antioxidant and anti-inflammatory action, thereby strengthening the immunological system. Blackcurrants help prevent the proliferation of the flu virus – much in the manner of elderberry (p. 100) – during the early stages of contraction.

Flavonoids found in both leaf and berry help fortify capillaries and peripheral circulation, making the tea a benefit to prevent/address arteriosclerosis, varicose veins, stroke and apoplexy, diabetic neuropathy, Raynaud's disease, aspects of dementia and erectile dysfunction. Utilised as a menopause support and rejuvenation tonic. The polyphenol phytochemicals stimulate digestion and also enhance the functioning of the liver, kidneys, spleen and pancreas.

Leaf infusions have a tradition in fighting fatigue and stress-related illnesses, and in adrenal support. Fruit infusions, on the other hand, have a reputation in improving daytime visual acuity and enhancing night vision.

Main medicinal actions: Anti-inflammatory, antioxidant, antiviral, detox, diaphoretic, digestive, diuretic, immunostimulant, ophthalmic, stress relief, vasoprotective.

Dosage

A daily cup delivers all the general benefits. Therapeutic dosages may stretch to 2–3 cups daily for the duration of treatment of a specific condition.

Caution

Generally regarded as safe, but prolonged use may enhance the effects of anticoagulants and interact with monoamine oxidase inhibitor (MAOI) medications.

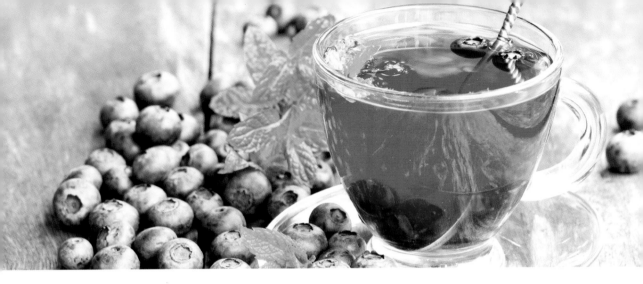

Blueberry Berry Tea

(Vaccinium corymbosum and V. angustifolium)

Botanical family
Ericaceae

Parts used
Fruit

Flavour profile
Sweet, tart

Blueberries are much lauded as a 'superfood' with a compelling antioxidant value and plenty of nutrients. There are several teas on the market with 'blueberry tea' written on the packaging, which are in fact a green or black 'blueberry-flavoured' tea, or a fruity mix of blueberries and other fruits, herbs and plant parts. This entry is for pure blueberry fruit tea.

How to make
There are many variations on the theme of how to make this particular tea, though it is mainly done via decoction. But I discount decoctions and boiling to a syrup base, as the heat can destroy many of the beneficial antioxidants contained in the fruit. I prefer a 4–10-minute infusion with 1-minute-rested boiled water – with either 1 tablespoon of quartered fresh berries or 1 teaspoon of chopped dried berry. The taste is milder than a sweet-tart berry but still in the range of sweet and sour. Teabag varieties are available but, as mentioned above, they are not always single ingredient and this can impact upon taste at longer steepage. Pleasant hot, or chilled to serve over ice.

Health benefits
Blueberries have a lot going on – especially when the berry is ingested, but much of the fruit's healing chemistry is water soluble so a herbal tea

is a great way to also include some of their health benefits into your day. The tea is a rich source of anthocyanidins (including cyanidin, delphinidin, malvidin, pelargonidins, peonidin and petunidin), which help to suppress several types of cancer cells (in particular cervical and colon lines) and help to lower blood cholesterol, reduce lipid peroxidation and support cognitive function and memory.

This tea is packed with vitamin C, which stimulates the production and activation of white blood cells. Its flavonols, such as quercetin, myricetin and kaempferol, have anti-inflammatory, anti-diabetic and more anticancer properties, as they disrupt the signalling pathways required for the proliferation and survival of cancer cells. Myricetin may also help restore dopamine levels and inhibit beta-amyloid fibril formation – two key issues with Alzheimer's, Parkinson's and other dementia illnesses.

Blueberries are rich in resveratrol – a polyphenolic phytoalexin created by some plants as a defence against pathogens. It is anti-microbial against a wide range of fungi and bacteria, which accounts for the berry's traditional relationship to stomach health and in fighting infections. When ingested by humans, resveratrol also reduces blood viscosity and inhibits platelet aggregation, thereby supporting cardiac health and venous integrity.

Blueberries also contain moderate levels of vitamin K, manganese and dietary fibre, as well as containing antioxidant anthocyanins, which are believed to increase communication between brain cells and hence may have a role to play in preventing age-related memory loss. Furthermore, the fruits also contain ellagic acid, which is considered to be potentially effective against cancer.

Main medicinal actions: Anticancer, anti-diabetic, anti-inflammatory, antimicrobial, antioxidant, antiviral, cognitive support, hypotensive, immune support, neuroprotective, vasodilation.

Dosage
1–3 cups daily.

Caution
Avoid if allergic to salicylates.

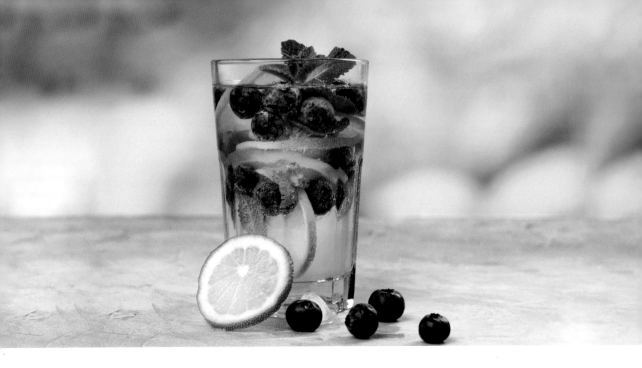

Blueberry Leaf Tea

(*Vaccinium corymbosum* and *V. angustifolium*)

Botanical family
Ericaceae

Parts used
Leaves

Flavour profile
Sweet, grassy

Blueberry foliage tea has a long folk history. Contemporary teabag and loose blueberry foliage tea may be acquired from most local health stores. Some brands may be a green tea mixed with blueberry foliage – this will thus be caffeinated and hold many of the actions of green tea. Blueberry foliage can be collected from the garden and dried as with standard herbs.

How to make
Some recipes call for a decoction, but as protracted exposure to heat impacts upon the phytochemistry, I prefer an infusion of 3–7 minutes utilising 1–2 teaspoons of chopped herb (fresh or dried) per cup. Longer brews can attain a stronger astringency but can be sweetened with stevia, honey or a fruit juice. Pleasant hot or iced.

Health benefits
We know that the blueberry fruit is a 'superfood', but it turns out that the foliage may be a superior beverage. This has nothing to do with taste and everything to do with its higher percentage of health-

conferring constituents. The foliage is filled with roughly thirty times more anthocyanins and antioxidants than the berries. That's thirty times more savaging of free radicals and thirty times more strengthening of capillaries and nerve endings.

The capillary strengthening action is of great benefit to slow the progression of diabetic neuropathy and retinopathy. The anthocyanins leached from the leaf can also help to lower excess blood glucose by improving insulin resistance and are protective of cells that make up the pancreas. Those same agents help reduce triglycerides (fats left over from excess calorie consumption found in the bloodstream and stored in fatty tissue) and so support cleaner arteries and promote cardiovascular health.

The high ratio of anthocyanins relates to a wide range of beneficial biological activities, including the inhibition of pro-inflammatory mediators connected not just to inflammation and pain perception/ signalling, but those that are also implicated in the initiation of degenerative diseases.

Blueberry leaf tea also has an application in balancing gut flora post antibiotics and in treating candida (a fungal infection that can arise in the mouth, stomach or vagina). Its antimicrobial nature makes it of use against urinary tract infections and it also contains ellagic acid, which undermines the capacity of bacteria to adhere to the walls of the bladder. Meanwhile, its content of ellagic and hippuric acids raise the acidity of urine, further diminishing bacteria's chances of surviving and replicating. Topical applications of the cooled tea also have a history in addressing eczema, psoriasis and other inflammatory skin diseases.

Main medicinal actions: Anticarcinogenic, anti-inflammatory, anti-oxidant, blood tonic, nervine, neuroprotective, vasoprotective.

Dosage
Therapeutic dosages are in the range of 1–2 cups daily – do not exceed 3–4 cups per day.

Caution
Over-consumption can potentially trigger hypoglycaemia (a drop in blood sugar levels to below normal range).

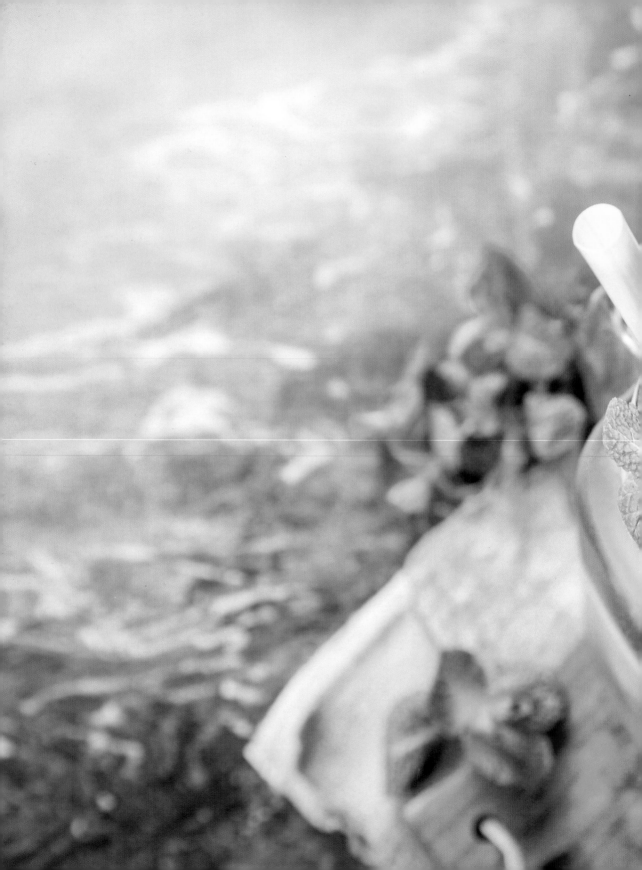

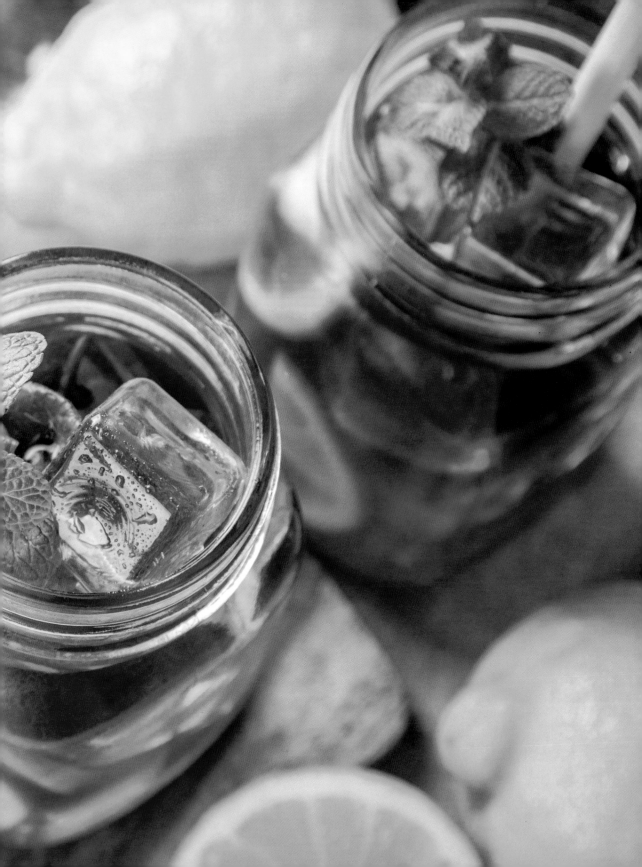

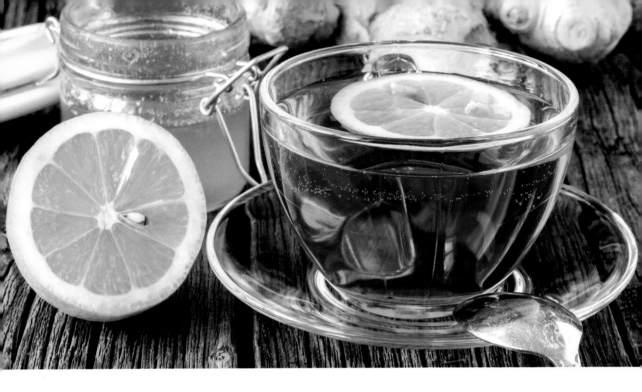

Burdock Tea

(*Arctium lappa*)

Botanical family
Asteraceae

Parts used
Roots and/or seeds
and leaves

Flavour profile
Sweet, earthy

Burdock is prized as a serious detoxifier and is often included in blends with dandelion or other detox herbs. Proprietary brands of burdock tea may feature a blend of seeds, dried leaves and dried root, but there is also a tradition of a simple tea comprised of fresh or dried root.

How to make
The traditional way is a decoction via a fast boil followed by simmering for 5–10 minutes – generally 2 teaspoons of herbage per cup required, with an extra half cup on hand to top up if too much liquid evaporates.

When it comes to a simple root tea, an infusion with freshly boiled water will suffice if given a 5–7-minute steepage time – use 1 teaspoon fresh/1–2 teaspoons dried/1 teabag. Can be sweetened to taste.

Health benefits
In traditional Chinese medicine, burdock is recommended to remedy intestinal worms and other parasites. Across many medicinal systems it is seen as the master detox herb and 'blood purifier'. It boosts

cellular metabolism, tones glandular functioning, activates digestion, stimulates liver and kidney function, supports lymphatic drainage, aids circulation and increases urine output and/or prompts sweating to expel toxins.

While popular as a bitter tonic to spring clean the system, it also has applications in the treatment of gout and rheumatoid arthritis; acne and psoriasis; to detox heavy metals (such as lead, mercury and arsenic) that can accumulate from environmental pollution and some cancer treatments; and to help break down calcification in the joints. It also has a reputation as a skin cleanser, but this is more as a topical treatment (administered to the skin, as one would a cosmetic treatment), as the detox process can actually aggravate skin conditions when toxins are sweated out, but this aggravation will resolve upon the ending of the treatment.

The chlorogenic acid found in the roots and leaves of burdock acts to regulate blood pressure and blood sugar levels, enhance circulation and also offers an anti-inflammatory effect. B1 and other vitamins and minerals in burdock tea support neurologic and memory function. Burdock root is also a pretty good source of polysaccharides, phenolic acids and sesquiterpene lactones, which are immunostimulants and which also exert many anticancer and antiviral effects. Arctiopicrin, a bitter glycoside in burdock, is antibiotic in action, while the inulin it contains is a probiotic.

Main medicinal actions: Antihelmintic, anti-inflammatory, antimicrobial, antimutagenic, bitter tonic, cholagogue, detox, diaphoretic, diuretic, hepatoprotective, hypoglycaemic, immunostimulant, laxative, probiotic.

Dosage
The potency restricts its use to short-burst treatments of 4–7 days with upper limits of 2–3 cups per day.

Caution
Not for long-term, recurrent use. Avoid if allergic to the daisy family. Avoid in pregnancy. May intensify the action of diabetic medications and interact with some prescription medications.

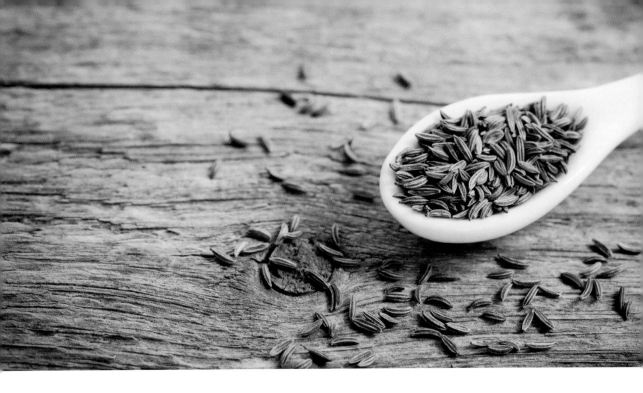

Caraway Tea

(Carum carvi)

Botanical family
Apiaceae

Parts used
Seeds

Flavour profile
Sweet, anise

Caraway was utilised as a culinary ingredient as far back as 3000 BC. Not only is it one of the oldest cultivated spices, but its medicinal value is prized in many of the earliest herbal codices for its ability to remedy gastric upset and as a mother's support (to hasten delivery of the placenta, recoup from labour strain, promote milk flow, etc.). The seed is actually the dried entire fruit. Caraway is often found in herbal tea blends as a flavour enhancer.

How to make
The standard recommendation is an infusion of 3–10 minutes. I would recommend letting the boiled water rest for almost a minute before making the infusion, which should preferably be made in a covered vessel in order to retain maximum volatile oils.

This is also available in teabags, or you can utilise store-bought seeds: 1 teaspoon per cup. To enrich flavour and allow more constituents to leach into the tea, crush the seed with the back of a spoon before infusing.

Health benefits

Caraway tea is a historic treatment for stimulating appetite, improving digestion and relieving flatulence. The rich array of volatile oils, including carvone and limonene, are antispasmodic – but with a caveat. A side effect is the relaxing of the oesophageal sphincter, which, if too relaxed, can increase the potential for reflux or heartburn. As a result, caraway is often blended with other herbs that counter that issue.

Traditionally utilised to treat intestinal parasites, stomach bugs and urinary tract infections, it can also help lower the concentration of LDL cholesterol and support the elimination of accumulated waste materials and toxins. As a diuretic and tonic, it also helps regulate the function of kidneys.

Caraway prompts breast-milk production and supports easier lactation. It also addresses colic and digestive upset in the nursing infant. It remains, in many regions around the world, a popular paediatric herb to treat cough, bronchitis and croup. For adults, it is often cooled and used as a gargle for tonsillitis and laryngitis.

The phytoestrogens in caraway can help regulate the menstrual cycle and reduce menstrual cramps. It is a source of iron and improves iron absorption, and is also a trace source of copper, which is utilised in red blood cell production, so is therefore beneficial for treating anaemia. The seeds also contain many B-complex vitamins and so this is considered a pick-me-up beverage.

Main medicinal actions: Analgesic, antioxidant, antispasmodic, carminative, digestive, emmenagogue, expectorant, febrifuge, galactagogue, oestrogenic.

Dosage

Generally 1–2 cups daily for treatment duration, upper limit of 2–3 cups daily. A daily cup as an iced tea can be sipped a little at a time at meal times.

Caution

Over-consumption can instigate nausea and a narcotic effect, including drowsiness and mental fog.

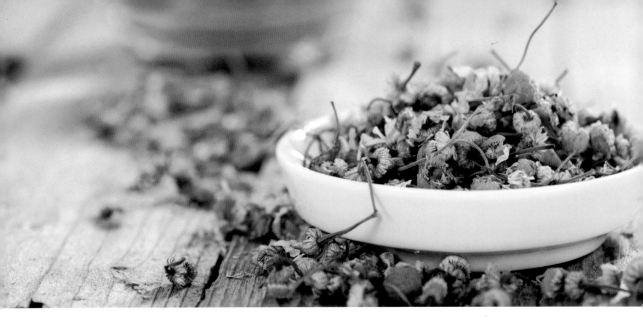

Chamomile Tea

(*Chamaemelum nobile* and *Matricaria recutita*)

Botanical family
Asteraceae

Parts used
Flowers

Flavour profile
Mildly sweet, floral

Chamomile is one of the oldest recorded therapeutic plants, stretching back to honourable mentions by the ancients of Greece, Rome, China and Egypt. There are several species of chamomile, but the two most utilised in ancient and modern herbalism are Roman Chamomile (*Chamaemelum nobile* syn. *Anthemis nobilis*) and German Chamomile (*Matricaria recutita*). They are used interchangeably. Some tea blends even combine both.

How to make
Standard infusion is of 3–5 minutes duration. Add a single teabag or 1–2 teaspoons of dried flowers to each cup required. Because the full flavour and medicinal actions are contained in the volatile oils of the plant, the tradition is to use hot water that has rested off the boil for 30–60 seconds. Cover the cup or put the lid on the teapot to maximise volatile oil retention. Chamomile tea has a very pleasant taste; its apple-like aroma overlies a mildly sweet, floral note.

Health benefits
Chamomile tea is well known as a night-time sedative and daytime antidepressant. It has shown great results with general anxiety,

insomnia and mild depression – in part due to the concentrations of apigenin, which bind to the benzodiazepine receptors in the brain in the same way Xanax and Valium do, but without the long-term side effects. Smelling the aroma of chamomile tea as you drink further reduces anxiety and tension, and promotes a sense of being refreshed – the aroma reduces levels of a certain hormone produced in response to biological and physical stresses.

Chamomile tea is also highly regarded as a treatment for all kinds of gastrointestinal disturbances – from digestive sluggishness and stomach cramps to the treatment of IBS and colitis. It helps relax muscle contractions, naturally cleanses the gut and promotes mineral absorption. It also contains constituents useful for the alleviation of rheumatic and muscular pain – in particular azulene and bisabolol, which are both potently anti-inflammatory and antispasmodic.

Chamomile has a long history in paediatric herbalism to treat colic, croup and fevers, and also to alleviate digestive upset, including diarrhoea. Topically applied, the cooled tea has application with skin irritations from eczema to nappy rash.

Main medicinal actions: Analgesic, anti-allergenic, antibacterial, anti-emetic, antihistamine, anti-inflammatory, antimicrobial, antiseptic, antispasmodic, anti-ulcer, anxiolytic, carminative, diaphoretic, digestive, diuretic, emmenagogue, hypnotic, nervine, uterine tonic, vulnerary.

Dosage

A daily cup is refreshing and remedial. Upper limits of 3–4 cups daily for supervised treatment durations. Consult a specialist for childhood applications.

Caution

Avoid if allergic to ragweed/daises. Upper limit doses can cause drowsiness. Regular use of chamomile can enhance the efficiency/action of certain medications, such as anticoagulants and antiplatelets, blood pressure and diabetes medications, sedatives, tricyclic antidepressants and benzodiazepines. Be cautious about use in early pregnancy due to uterine interaction.

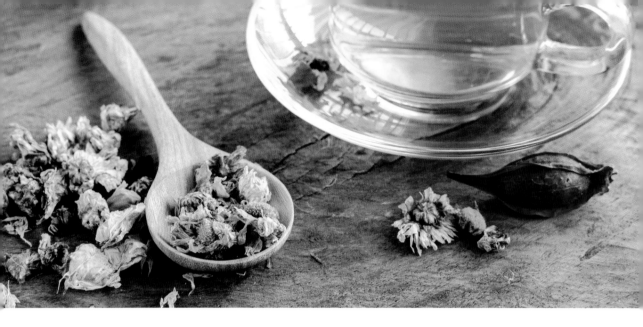

Chrysanthemum Tea

(Chrysanthemum morifolium and C. indicum)

Botanical family
Asteraceae

Parts used
Flowers/flower buds

Flavour profile
Floral, sweet

There are approximately 100 species of chrysanthemum, some with potent insecticidal and toxin chemistry. The edible/medical source is generally one of two: *Chrysanthemum morifolium* or *Chrysanthemum indicum*. While there is such a thing as chrysanthemum pu-erh (a mix of flowers and true tea), this entry refers to pure, non-adulterated chrysanthemum tea.

How to make
While there are various traditions around chrysanthemum tea and suggestions to infuse at varying temperatures – generally in the range of 90°C (194°F) to 95°C (203°F) – a kettle rested off the boil for 30–60 seconds will be sufficient. A single teabag or a single rounded teaspoon or 4–5 dried flowers per cup required is the ratio. The infusion duration is 3–5 minutes, covered. Works well hot or as iced tea – the flavour is a slightly sweet, floral tone. Can be further sweetened to taste.

Health benefits
Chrysanthemum tea is refreshing and reviving, popular as a body coolant for fever or prickly heat and as a convalescence beverage for flu, viruses, colds and chest infections. In traditional Chinese medicine

it was often suggested for longevity and to treat/clear the liver, to improve vision and to remedy hypertension and angina. In Japan it was recommended to regulate blood pressure, clear and strengthen lungs, and in relieving sinusitis congestion. In Korea it is viewed as a pick-me-up, skin treatment, detox and headache relief.

Packed with potent flavonoids such as luteolin, apigenin and acacetin, as well as a range of minerals and vitamins that make it beneficial to cancer prevention and potential co-therapy (used in conjunction with conventional treatments). Luteolin, which is studied for its anti-tumour properties, also exerts a strong anti-inflammatory and potent antioxidant action to scavenge reactive compounds containing oxygen and nitrogen, thus restricting cellular damage. Apigenin and acacetin show promise with breast and prostate cancer inhibition respectively. Chrysanthemum tea is also anti-spirochetal and may have good application in unwinding spirochetal (corkscrew-like bacterial) conditions from their embedded nature in tissues, thereby aiding with the treatment of conditions such leptospirosis and Lyme disease.

Main medicinal actions: Analgesic, antibacterial, anti-infective, anti-inflammatory, antioxidant, anti-spirochetal, anti-tumour, antiviral, chemoprotective, circulatory support, coolant, digestive, detox, hypotensive, immunostimulant, nervine, restorative.

Dosage

Recommendations rarely exceed 1 cup daily for the duration of the remedy. Iced chrysanthemum tea is a popular beverage worldwide. Once thought of as a summer tea, which therefore meant there was a limit to intake, that limit is now regularly surpassed and so, due to the cautions listed below, I would advise supervision or guidance if taking for prolonged periods. Also beware of the fact that many commercial iced teas are loaded with sugar and sweeteners.

Caution

Avoid in pregnancy. Avoid if you are allergic to ragweed. Because of its immunostimulant potential, chrysanthemum tea is not recommended in instances of autoimmune diseases. Prolonged use can potentially increase photosensitivity in some.

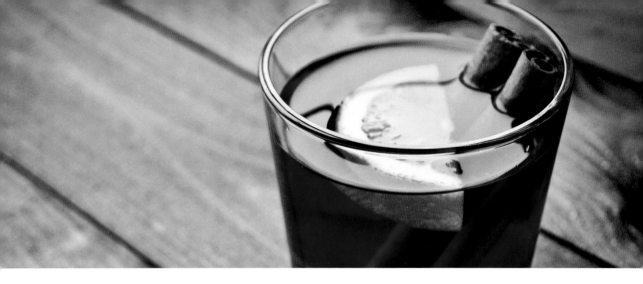

Cinnamon Tea

(*Cinnamomum verum* and *C. cassia*)

Botanical family
Lauraceae

Parts used
Inner bark (quills)
or ground spice

Flavour profile
Sweet, spicy

Cinnamon is derived from the inner bark of any of several species of tree defined as a cinnamon tree, and while there are many, the two most prominent in culinary and medicinal circles are Ceylon cinnamon (*Cinnamomum verum*), also known as 'true cinnamon', and Chinese cinnamon (*Cinnamomum cassia*), also known as 'Cassia spice'.

How to make
Traditionally, these teas are made from the quills or spice. Teabag versions are also often available, but may contain extra ingredients. Cinnamon is often utilised as a sweetener to other herbal teas. The preferred means of making this tea is to decoct a finger-length quill in 2 cups of water. Start from cold, bring to a simmering boil for 2 minutes and rest off the heat for 10–15 minutes. Reheat, if required, before straining and serving. Second brews from the same quill are possible. It is generally taken that 1 quill equals 1 teaspoon of ground spice. Alternatively, infuse for 4–5 minutes in boiling water at a ratio of 1 teaspoon per cup. Teabag infusions are best in the range of 3–7 minutes.

Health benefits
Traditionally, this tea is consumed to speed convalescence or prevent chronic diseases. Its gastroprotective nature comes via strongly

antibacterial and antifungal actions. Cinnamon relaxes muscles and alleviates spasms, while lessening indigestion and cramping. It is also packed with water soluble polyphenols that actively inhibit the oxidative processes known as peroxidation – the process whereby fats and lipids are changed into inflammatory compounds rather than metabolised.

Cinnamon mimics an insulin-like biological activity and enhances insulin signalling, improving glucose control and helping to slow/prevent insulin resistance. The role of cinnamon as a circulatory tonic may address diabetic neuropathy. One of the compounds within cinnamon – cinnamaldehyde – supplies hypotensive and anticoagulant actions supportive to vascular and cardiac health.

Cinnamon charts with an oxygen radical absorbance capacity rating many hundred times more potent than apples, blueberries and other 'superfoods' – hence its promotion of improved cognitive function and alertness. It is metabolised by the body into sodium benzoate, which acts to prevent the loss of two neuroprotective proteins – DJ-1 and Parkin – both of which are vital in maintaining healthy neurotransmitter levels in the brain and which are implicated in slowing the progression of Parkinson's disease.

Main medicinal actions: Analgesic, anti-inflammatory, antimicrobial, antispasmodic, appetite stimulant, astringent, carminative, digestive, gastroprotective, hypoglycaemic, hypotensive, neuroprotective, stimulant, styptic, vascular tonic.

Dosage
Generally confined to ½–1 teaspoon per day (equivalent to 2–4g ground spice) or a single cup per day. Cassia for short-term usage only.

Caution
Avoid with liver disease. Recurrent use may interact with some prescription medications. The blood-thinning and often health problematic coumarin content is only found in cassia not verum and, as it is not water-soluble, quills are safe, but coumarin will be ingested via ground spice tea.

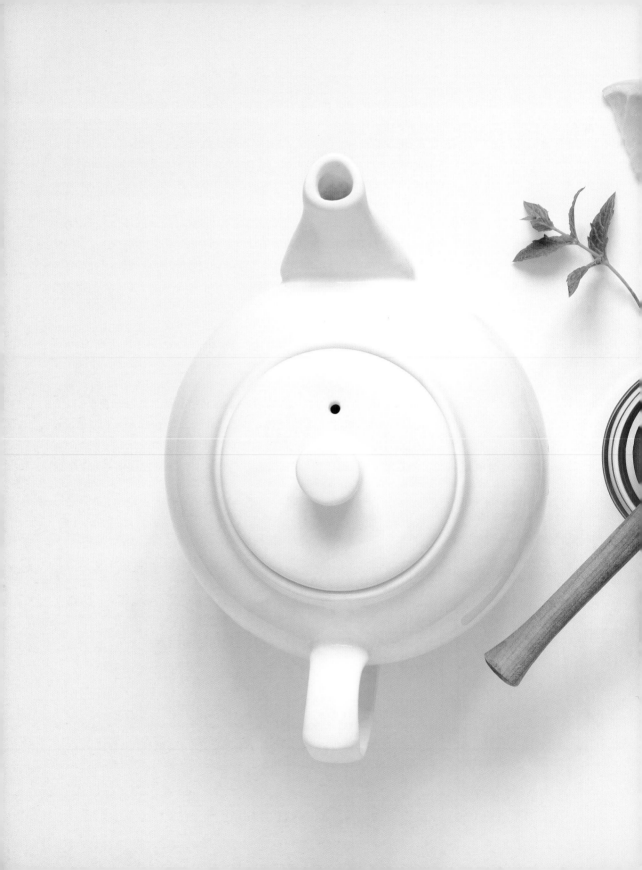

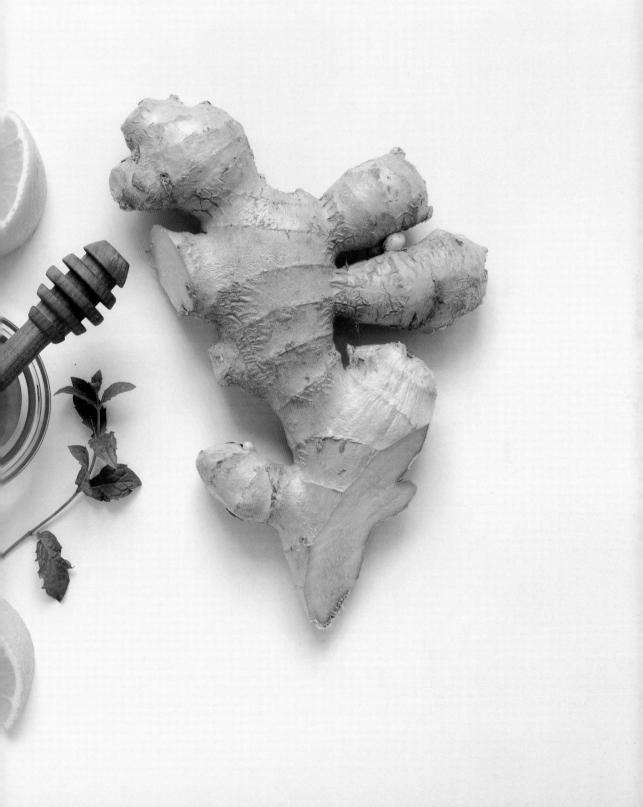

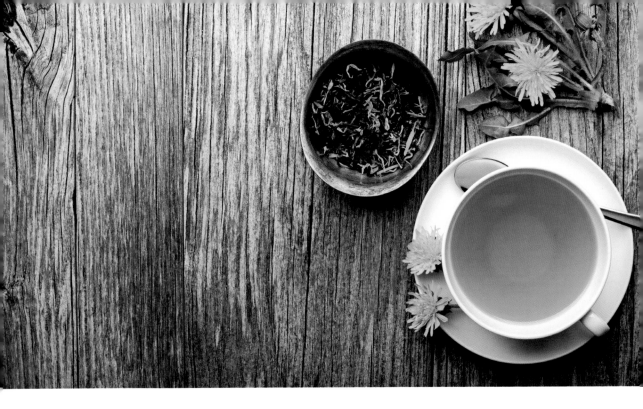

Dandelion Leaf Tea

(*Taraxacum officinale*)

Botanical family
Asteraceae

Parts used
Foliage

Flavour profile
Bitter

From the French for the lion's tooth – *dent-de-lion* – the large-toothed leaves are noticeably serrated and they also pack a medicinal bite with some potent bitter glycosides, terpenoids and a good complement of vitamins and minerals, including plenty of potassium and iron. Dandelion leaf is sold in loose form in health stores and in teabags in many places. Some dandelion tea brands mix the leaf with other herbs or green tea and so include additional medicinal actions. It is also available from the garden (if you happen to own one, even a neglected one) to use fresh, or can be dried for later use.

How to make
The tradition is for a dried leaf infusion, utilising 1–2 teaspoons of chopped herbage per cup of boiling water (a similar ratio applies for fresh herbage). Steep for 3–7 minutes. The fresh foliage is slightly less bitter than the dried. Both will attain more astringency with longer soakage. Both can be sweetened to improve taste.

Health benefits

Dandelion foliage exerts a strong diuretic action, increasing the amount of urine production and stimulating urination, and so has a long history in treating urinary tract infections, oedema, high blood pressure and glaucoma, and to eliminate uric acid and as a detox. Unlike conventional diuretics, which cause a loss of potassium, dandelion tea contains good levels of potassium.

A traditional spring tonic, its bitter agents known as glycosides, including taraxacin and taraxacerin, can ease the symptoms and flare-ups of arthritis, acne, eczema and gastritis. The herb is often utilised as a cleanser of the kidney, spleen, gall bladder and liver. Dandelion leaf also increases bile production and stomach acids, stimulating the appetite and assisting efficient digestion. It is a potent source of kynurenic acid, which plays a role in the healthy functioning of the digestive system and gut flora, and is remedial to diseases of the gastrointestinal tract.

It is naturally rich in antioxidants that prevent free-radical damage to cells and help slow breakdown of DNA strands and of cancer growth. It is packed with sesquiterpene lactones and triterpene steroids (including sitosterin, stigmasterin and phytosterin), which show strong actions against inflammation and the development of certain cancers. The phenolic and polysaccharide content supports general well-being and, coupled with the vitamin C content, are supportive to illness prevention and recovery.

Main medicinal actions: Anti-inflammatory, antibacterial, bitter tonic, chemopreventive, cholagogue, detox, digestive, diuretic.

Dosage

Therapeutic doses rarely exceed 2–3 cups daily.

Caution

Avoid if allergic to ragweed. May cancel the action of prescription antacids and increase the action of diuretics, diabetic medication and blood-thinning medications. As with all strong diuretics, anyone utilising lithium or with kidney or gall bladder problems will require guidance/supervision of use.

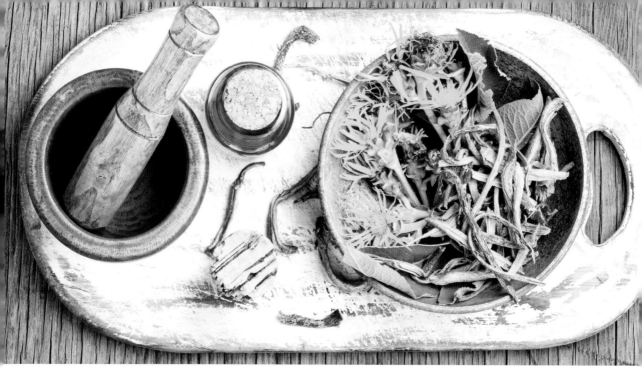

Dandelion Root Tea

(*Taraxacum officinale*)

Botanical family
Asteraceae

Parts used
Roots

Flavour profile
Bitter

Dandelion root is readily available in teabag form and as a loose herb. Roasted roots are often sold as a coffee substitute and do have a coffee-like flavour.

How to make
Dandelion root (dried or fresh) is traditionally decocted in boiling water for 5–10 minutes. The ratio is ½–2 teaspoons per cup, depending on preferred strength. Higher dosages are more potent therapeutically but also stronger in bitterness. Sweeten to taste.

Health benefits
The bitter principle and diuretic nature of dandelion root means it was traditionally availed of as an alternative for chronic toxin-related conditions such as arthritis, rheumatism, gout, eczema, acne, chronic gastritis and enteritis. It has a history of use as a cleanser of the kidney, spleen, gall bladder and liver. The tea helps remove excess uric acid and other toxin build-ups.

We have a 'bitter taste' receptor known as T2R38, which is implicated in upper respiratory infection and chronic rhinosinusitis, and the aroma of a bitter brew can fire up our anti-inflammatory radar if not actively engage our immune arsenal. Therefore, a bitter sup of dandelion root tea may be as beneficial to allergies as the immunology of local honey.

Like the leaves, the roots contain sesquiterpene lactones (including eudesmanolide and germacranolide), which act as anti-inflammatories. These also support the activity of the pancreas, and dandelion root contains two substances – inulin and levulin – that, as soluble fibres, can help reduce blood cholesterol, lower glucose levels and may see useful application in metabolic syndrome and diabetes treatments.

The levels of quercetin and various flavonoids available via a brew of dandelion root further exert anti-inflammatory, anti-allergenic and anti-diabetic actions. In supporting stimulation of bile flow from the gall bladder to the duodenum, dandelion helps to prompt the efficient digestion of fats and can be utilised to support detoxing from a former fatty diet. It is also considered a natural liver detox.

The diuretic nature is beneficial in treating hypertension and oedema. It also has a mild laxative effect, which will provide relief from constipation. Regular consumption of dandelion root tea also supports a reduction in total cholesterol, triglycerides and bad LDL cholesterol, and is supportive of an increase in beneficial HDL cholesterol.

Main medicinal actions: Anti-allergenic, anti-diabetic, anti-inflammatory, anti-rheumatic, bitter tonic, cholagogue, depurative, detox, digestive, diuretic, laxative, tonic.

Dosage
A daily cup is health bolstering. Therapeutic dosages tend to remain within the limits of 3 times daily for treatment duration.

Caution
Avoid if allergic to Asteraceae plants. May interact with diabetic and blood-thinning medications. As with all strong diuretics, anyone utilising lithium or with kidney or gall bladder problems will require guidance/ supervision of use.

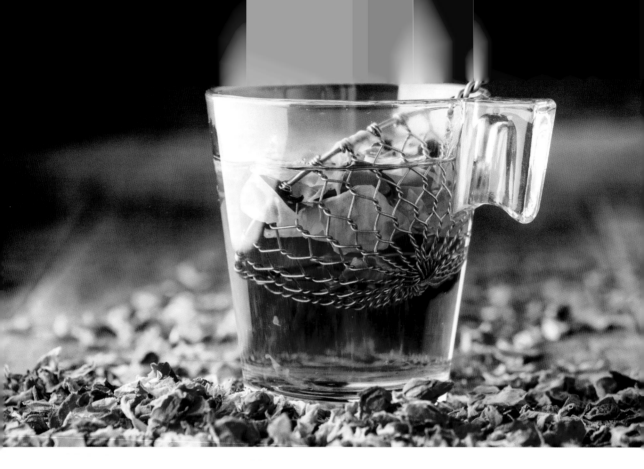

Echinacea Leaf and Cone Tea

(Echinacea angustifolia, E. purpurea and E. pallida)

Botanical family
Asteraceae

Parts used
Foliage and cones

Flavour profile
Bitter

Echinacea is sometimes referred to by the name 'cone flower' – a nod to the central cone of its flower, which develops into the seed head. The root is popularly employed in herbalism, but a tea of its foliage and seed heads makes a less bitter brew with many similar attributes.

How to make

Harvested from the garden or purchased ready dried from select health stores. The leaf and seed tea is best via a standard 3–5-minute infusion of 1–2 teaspoons of dried herbage per cup, or double if utilising fresh parts. Longer steepage may increase bitterness. Sweeten to taste.

Health benefits

The foliage and seed heads of echinacea contain compounds that exert potent immunological properties. Some in particular (glycosides and polysaccharides) encourage macrophage activation and phagocytosis – that's where white blood cells gobble up invading microorganisms. This munching up is how our immune system breaks them down and removes them from our system. The tea may take 4–7 days to kick in and some colds are over before activation happens, but with longer flu and other viral complaints this type of powerful immune system stimulation will be beneficial in reducing illness duration.

The presence of echinacein and cichoric acid also makes it quite effective against herpes simplex and flu, as these agents work by disrupting the integrase enzymes that facilitate how viruses invade cells. Echinacea's thermogenic (temperature raising) nature and the hot beverage delivery increases the body's core temperature and facilitates the body's other innate means of dealing with invading organisms – i.e. heat and sweating.

Echinacea tea stimulates an increased production of hyaluronic acid, which is not only a component of cartilage and synovial fluid, but is utilised to effect repairs at sites damaged by excessive inflammation markers or standard injury. Topically, the cooled tea is a great anti-microbial wound cleaner and healer.

Main medicinal actions: antibiotic, anti-catarrhal, anti-inflammatory, antimicrobial, antioxidant, anti-tumour, decongestant, depurative, dia-phoretic, immunostimulant, lymphatic, peripheral vasodilator, vulnerary.

Dosage

Not a long-term use tea and more reserved for treatment blocks – with 'on/off' periods of 5 days on and 5 off in order to maintain its potency. Generally 1–2 cups per day.

Caution

Avoid if allergic to ragweed. Avoid with autoimmune diseases, as raised white blood count is not beneficial. Echinacea can potentially interfere with immunosuppressant medication, steroids and other prescription medications.

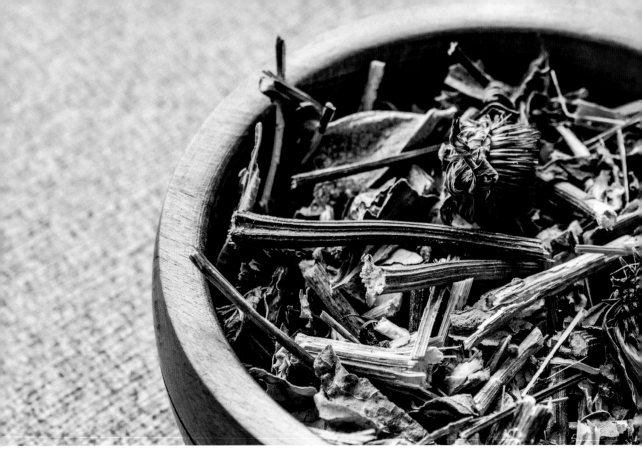

Echinacea Root Tea

(Echinacea angustifolia and *E. purpurea)*

Botanical family
Asteraceae

Parts used
Roots

Flavour profile
Strong, bitter

Echinacea is grown all over the world as an ornamental garden plant and as a medicinal herb. It is a native of North America and had a long ethnobotanical tradition as an antibiotic, wound healer and tonic among many of the Great Plains tribes before its introduction to European herbalism.

How to make
The flavour molecules and plant chemistry of roots are always best extracted via a decoction. Traditionally the dried root would be simmered for 15–20 minutes. The standard ratio is 1g of herb per cup required. The root is quite bitter and will need sweetening with honey or other sweetener. Teabag versions are generally infused in hot water for 3–7 minutes.

Health benefits

The prime constituents of echinacea roots include polysaccharides, glycoproteins and glycosides, all of which stimulate or support white blood cell activations, thereby increasing our natural defence against viral invasion and disease manifestation. Echinacea also improves the efficiency of T-cells, which seek and destroy abnormal cells, including cancer cells. Echinacea also induces the release of tumour necrosis factor, which tackles cancer cell lines.

The roots also contain high proportions of alkamides and poly-acetylenes. Polyacetylenes are natural immunostimulants with noted antibacterial and antifungal actions. Similarly alkamides are antibacterial and antifungal and also help in the boosting of immune function and signalling. Alkamides also have an effect on the cannabinoid receptor type 2, which has some immunomodulatory function but is also anti-inflammatory via the inhibition of both COX 1 and COX 2 and 5-lipoxygenase.

Echinacea root is much lauded as a potent antiviral and many trials have found the plant chemistry effective against the seasonal influenza pathogen (H3N2), as well as H5N1 (avian), H7N7 (bird) and H1N1 (swine) flus. It also reduces respiratory syncytial virus and herpes simplex. Not only does echinacea help our immune system gobble up the invaders, but it also interferes with their ability to replicate and adhere to cell walls.

Main medicinal actions: Antibiotic, anti-catarrhal, anti-inflammatory, anti-microbial, antioxidant, anti-tumour, decongestant, depurative, diaphoretic, immunostimulant, lymphatic, peripheral vasodilator, vulnerary.

Dosage

Best in short-term use – reserved for treatment blocks with 'on/off' periods of 5 days on and 5 off so as to maintain its potency. Generally 1–2 cups per day.

Caution

Avoid if allergic to ragweed. Avoid with autoimmune diseases, as raised white blood count is not beneficial. Echinacea can potentially interfere with immunosuppressant medication, steroids and other prescription medications of similar or contra medicinal attributes to itself.

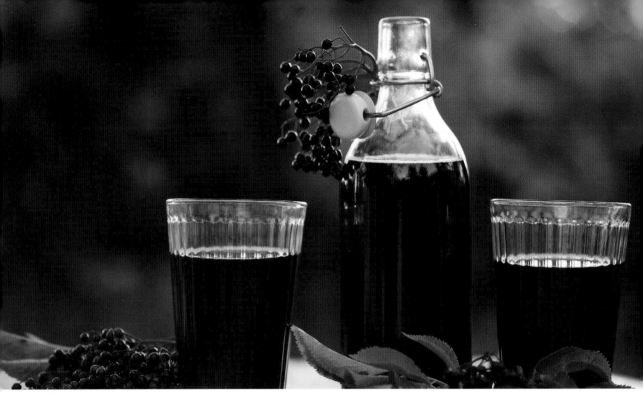

Elderberry Tea

(Sambucus nigra)

Botanical family
Adoxaceae

Parts used
Dried berries

Flavour profile
Tart

Elderberry is one of the most foraged and easily recognisable medicinal plants. If you are foraging the fruits, please note that the seeds within raw elderberries contain some glycosides with unpleasant side effects (emetic, purgative, potentially cyanide-inducing) and so need to be destroyed by cooking/heat or a drying process before consumption. The extra benefit of this process is that exposure to heat concentrates the bioavailable levels of elderberry's polyphenols and anthocyanins – wherein lie the bulk of its medicinal actions.

How to make
Older traditions involved decocting 1–2 teaspoons of pierced berry per cup, simmered for 30 minutes, then rested for 10 minutes before straining and serving. Today, dried berries (which are diminished of glycosides in their processing) are suitable for a 5–10-minute decoction, or an infusion via boiling water for 3–7 minutes. Teabag versions can be infused in hot water for 3–7 minutes. Elderberry tea is quite tart –

sweeten to taste. Some proprietary brands may contain additional ingredients.

Health benefits

Traditionally utilised for treating respiratory disorders from bronchitis to the common cold, it is particularly useful in cases of sinusitis via the reduction of excessive mucus secretion and nasal passage inflammation/irritation. It also supports better sinus drainage. Its anti-microbial action wards off bacterial and viral infections at the root of certain respiratory problems.

Its antiviral potency has seen it heralded as a 'flu buster', as the berry flavonoids don't just boost the immune system response to infection, but actually bind to flu strains and lessen their potential to grip onto cell structures and take hold. It is possible to reduce the duration of a cold or flu by several days by limiting its spread through the system. The berries are also full of *Sambucus nigra* agglutinin (SNA), a lectin that coats the sialic acid structures of viruses, putting an extra barrier between the cell wall and the hooks of the virus. SNA also binds to sialic acid structures on ovarian cancer cells and inhibits both their movement and growth. Because metastatic cancer cells have a much higher formation of sialic acid structures than other cells, there is potential in a 'pharma grade' elderberry agglutinin as a line of future treatment.

Main medicinal actions: Analgesic, adaptogen, anti-inflammatory, anti-microbial, antioxidant, antiviral, astringent, decongestant, diaphoretic, diuretic, febrifuge, immunostimulant, laxative, relaxant.

Dosage

The accepted protocol is between 1–3 cups daily for durations of 5 days followed by a 2-day rest and a resumption cycle until treatment duration is complete.

Caution

Avoid in pregnancy. May undermine corticosteroids and medications used to treat autoimmune diseases. May increase the effects of diabetic medication.

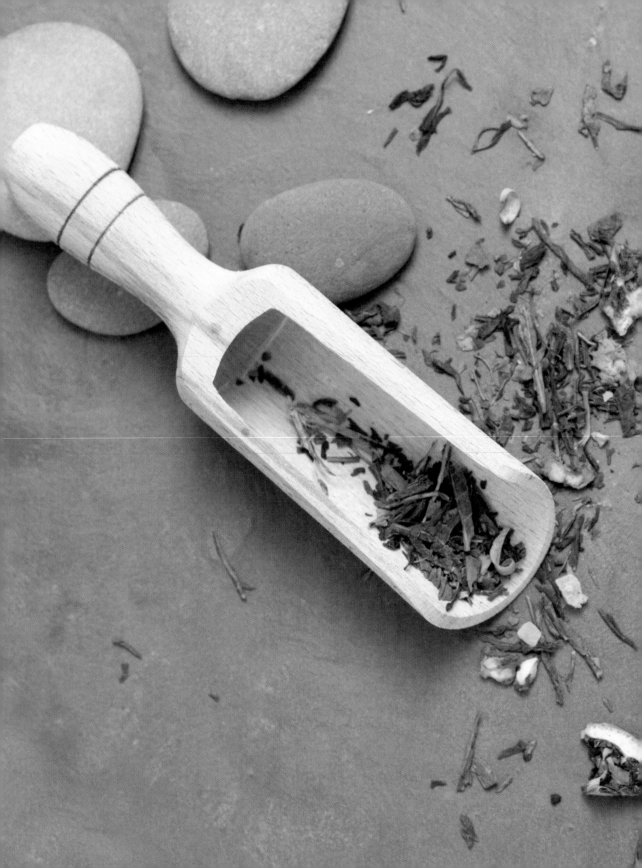

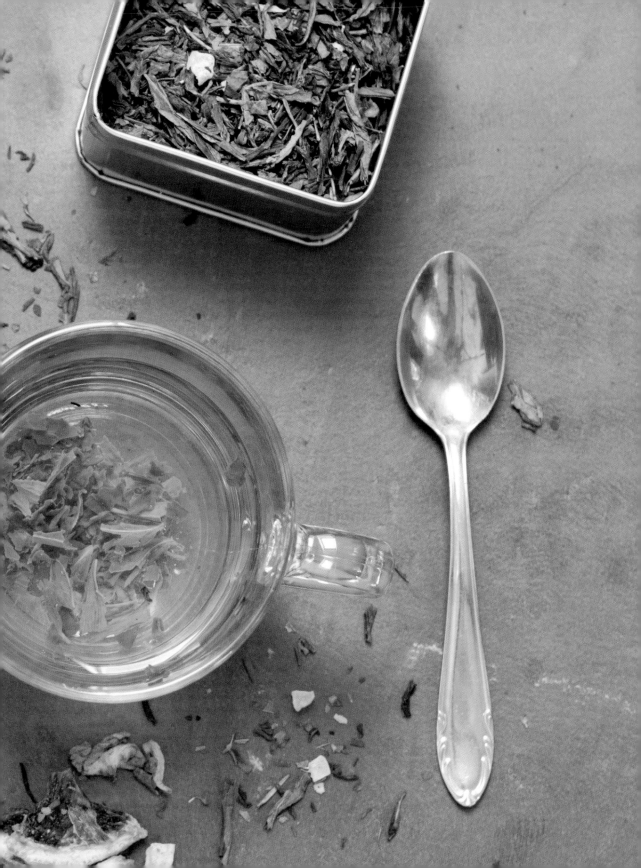

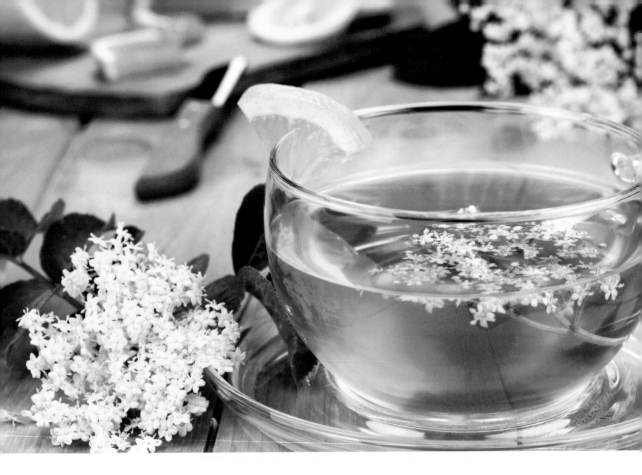

Elderflower Tea

(*Sambucus nigra*)

<u>Botanical family</u>
Adoxaceae

<u>Parts used</u>
Dried flowers

<u>Flavour profile</u>
Slightly sweet, floral

Elderflower tea is a fine herbal tea in its own right. Dried elderberry flowers are available in select health stores. Proprietary blends of elderflower tea frequently have additional ingredients, often including other immune system-boosting herbs. Elderflower tea has many of the attributes of elderberry tea and sometimes they can feature together in a blend.

How to make

My personal preference is for a longish infusion of 7–15 minutes, using off the boil water. However, some recipes and some teabag directions call for a faster 3–7-minute infusion via boiling water. The flower heads have a muscat/musky fragrance that imparts into the brew, so while there is a nuance of sweetness there can also be varying notes – the longer soak extracts more of the flavour. The tradition is 1–2 table-spoons of dried flowers per cup.

Health benefits

Packed with anti-allergenic flavonols, including quercetin and iso-quercetin, and popularly utilised to alleviate coughs, catarrh, bronchial congestion, asthma, croup, rhinitis, hay fever and histamine intolerance, and as a natural prophylactic to colds and flu. Quercetin and isoquercetin are known to significantly reduce the replication of flu viruses.

The combination of the herb's anti-inflammatory and febrifuge (fever-lowering) actions certainly help take the edge off aches, pains and fevers. It is also helpful to inflammatory conditions, including joint pain. It contains some plant chemicals called triterpenoids that are pain-relieving and vasorelaxant, and so can contribute to cardiac and vascular health, as well as help calm physical and mental tension or stress.

Elderflower tea is also a popular choice to alleviate the symptoms of digestive disorders and can mitigate bacterial-induced diarrhoea, constipation (it's mildly laxative at higher doses), indigestion, heartburn and queasiness. So effective is its antimicrobial action that elder extracts have been successfully tested for treating dangerous hospital pathogens, including MRSA.

Main medicinal actions: Adaptogen, anti-allergenic, anti-inflammatory, antimicrobial, antioxidant, astringent, carminative, decongestant, diaphoretic, diuretic, febrifuge, immunostimulant, relaxant, vasorelaxant.

Dosage

The standard is 1 cup daily for general health usage, graduating to 1–2 cups daily to treat specific conditions for the duration of the illness or flare-up.

Caution

Generally regarded as safe, but recurrent use or overuse can increase the actions of diabetes and blood-pressure medication. As with any herbal tea, excessive use may cause gastrointestinal upset.

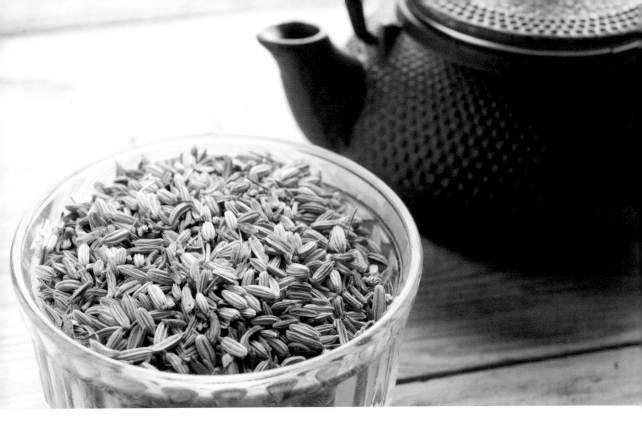

Fennel Tea

(Foeniculum vulgare)

Botanical family
Umbelliferae

Parts used
Seeds

Flavour profile
Anise-like

The ancient Greek name for the aromatic herb fennel was 'marathon' meaning 'to grow thin' – a nod to the stem structure and perhaps also to its ethnobotany, i.e. how people have traditionally utilised it for metabolism and weight management.

How to make
To extract the maximum phytochemicals, and thus the strongest benefits, it is best to crush the fennel seeds with the back of a spoon and then infuse in freshly boiled water for a period of 7–10 minutes. The standard ratio is 1–2 teaspoons per cup required to suit taste. The more seeds the stronger the anise/liquorice flavour. It is good to cover the tea cup or brew in a teapot. Can be sweetened to taste.

Health benefits
A long-standing remedy for upset stomach and digestive complaints

such as indigestion, heartburn, flatulence, etc. Fennel helps to neutralise excess acids in the stomach and calms cramping in the intestines. It helps promote a more efficient digestion and improves absorption of nutrients. As to its reputation in weight loss, beyond its ability to support the transition of food into energy rather than into stored fat, fennel may also curb appetite.

As an antispasmodic, it has form with menstrual cramps and also in the relief of bronchial spasms, asthma and seasonal allergies. It is not only a vasodilator (opening blood vessels and allowing blood to flow more easily), but contains many antihistamines, including quercetin, rutin and kaempferol glycosides. Fennel is a constituent of many cough remedies.

Its antispasmodic action combined with its galactagogue (pro-breast milk) potential means that it not only supports lactation in nursing mothers and remedies their digestive upset, but via its transition through breast milk helps remedy indigestion and colic in feeding babies. Fennel tea is a popular diuretic to address fluid retention in the body and also to help eliminate toxins. It has application as a detox tea, and also in the alleviation of arthritis and gout via the expulsion of excess uric acid.

Because fennel also exhibits antiseptic properties, it is utilised against urinary tract infections and is beneficial in treating cystitis, stones and gravel. Externally, cooled fennel tea can be utilised as an eyewash for conjunctivitis and as a soothing rinse for sore eyes.

Main medicinal actions: Antibacterial, antiemetic, antifungal, anti-inflammatory, anti-neuroinflammatory, antispasmodic, antitussive, aperient, carminative, digestive, diuretic, expectorant, galactagogue, oestrogenic, ophthalmic.

Dosage

½–1 cup at meal times for duration of treatment for gastrointestinal ailments. 1 cup daily for general consumption or other conditions.

Caution

Its weak oestrogenic effect often flags it as not suitable for use in cases of oestrogen dominance or oestrogen-related cancers.

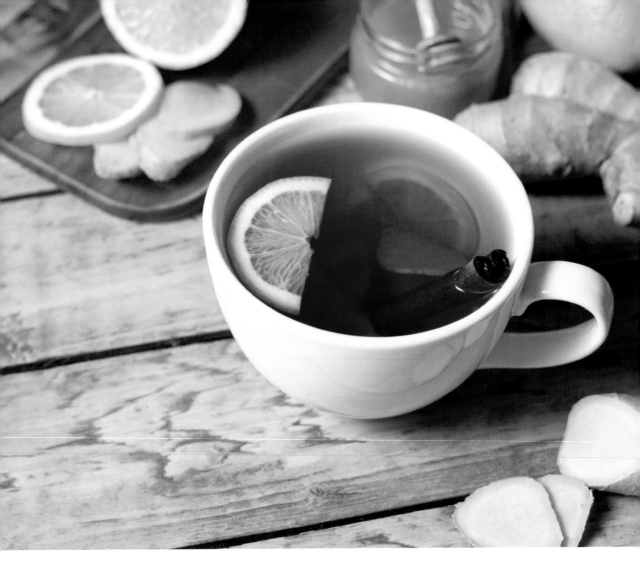

Ginger Tea

(Zingiber officinale)

Botanical family
Zingiberaceae

Parts used
Roots

Flavour profile
Peppery with lemony undertones

Ginger has a long history of culinary and medicinal use, and a long list of actions. It features in almost all medicinal systems, notably in Chinese, Indian, Arabic and Western herbal traditions. It is a popular go-to tea when it comes to health enhancement.

How to make
Traditionally ginger tea was brewed via a decoction – boiling or simmering fresh or dried root for 3–5 minutes at a rough ratio of 25–

30g root to 250–300ml water. Today there are teabag options and also powdered spice or shredded dried root that can be infused in boiled water. Dried root at a ratio of 1 teaspoon per cup required, ground spice at ⅓ teaspoon. As some of the main actions are down to volatile oils, making it in a teapot prevents evaporation, and waiting for the boiled water to cool a little will also keep more of them intact.

Health benefits

Ginger is warming and stimulating and is often utilised to take the edge off a cold or flu. It helps mitigate coughs and clears phlegm. Its content of gingerols and shogaols act in a similar manner to nonsteroidal anti-inflammatory drugs and also exert antispasmodic and analgesic actions. Ginger tea may be employed in relief of headache, period pains, muscle aches and intestinal cramps. Gingerols and shogaols can also moderate the effects of nausea and motion sickness.

Ginger tea is a popular remedy for sluggish digestion and to treat a variety of stomach upsets. It increases saliva production and encourages bile flow and the actions of digestive enzymes. It has applications in illnesses such as arthritis, too, where improved toxin elimination is beneficial.

Main medicinal actions: Analgesic, antibiotic, antiemetic, anti-inflammatory, antioxidant, antiseptic, antispasmodic, anti-thrombotic, antitussive, carminative, cholagogue, diaphoretic, digestive, emmenagogue, expectorant, gastrointestinal stimulant, hepatoprotective, hypotensive, immune support, peripheral circulatory stimulant, rubefacient, thermogenic, vasodilator.

Dosage

A daily cup delivers many benefits, while therapeutic dosages are in the range of 2–4 cups daily for set treatment duration.

Caution

Avoid with gallstones and peptic ulcers. Can increase the actions of medications prescribed for diabetes, blood pressure and blood-thinning. May reduce iron absorption. Ginger contains salicylates.

Ginkgo Tea

(Ginkgo biloba)

Botanical family
Ginkgoaceae

Parts used
Leaves

Flavour profile
Bittersweet

Ginkgo biloba is one of the earliest evolved trees to still survive today – the fossil record dates its existence back to the Permian period, roughly 299 to 251 million years ago. No wonder, then, that it is considered a longevity herb.

How to make
The tradition is a 4–7-minute infusion of 1–2 teaspoons of chopped herb per cup. Boiling water is fine for the dried herb, momentarily rested off the boil for the fresh leaf. Longer steepage can strengthen astringency (generally a bittersweet taste), but it can be flavoured with lemon and honey.

Health benefits
The earliest recorded medicinal uses of ginkgo date back 5000 years to China and remedies for asthma, allergies and respiratory complications. Ginkgo supplies seven antihistaminic phytochemicals and a dozen or more anti-inflammatory agents, as well as bronchodilation and antispasmodic actions – but it is perhaps the PAF link that is most interesting. PAF, or platelet-activating factor, is a pro-inflammatory mediator in the human system. Amongst other things it is reactive to allergens and is implicated in asthma. The unique chemicals found in

ginkgo plant parts, known as ginkgolides, strongly inhibit PAF formation and activity. PAF implicated conditions include acrocyanosis,
Raynaud's disease, peripheral vascular disease, cardiovascular
disease, erectile dysfunction, atherosclerosis, cerebral atherosclerosis,
Alzheimer's disease, dementia, senility, cochlear deafness, tinnitus,
vertigo, PMS, menopause, chronic fatigue, fibromyalgia, retinopathy
including glaucoma, depression and stress, and a whole plethora of
immune and inflammatory diseases.

Ginkgo flavonoids are powerfully antioxidant and reduce inflammation, engage immune responses and tone capillary function,
improving micro-circulation and healthier nerve-cell functions.
Ginkgo supports vascular dilation and blood flow, stabilises capillary
permeability, and increases oxygen and glucose uptake and utilisation.
All of this serves as neuroprotection, but the improved glucose uptake
by brain cells may be the mechanism behind ginkgo's reputation as an
improver of cognitive function and reliever of depression and anxiety.

Certainly ginkgo has been shown to attenuate stress-elevated
alterations in brain chemistry – notably with catecholamines, serotonin and corticosterone levels. These properties in ginkgo act as
monoamine oxidase inhibitors (MAOIs) in a similar way to many
prescription medications for depression and anxiety.

Main medicinal actions: Anti-allergenic, anti-asthmatic, antidepressant, anti-inflammatory, antioxidant, antiplatelet, antispasmodic,
anti-thrombotic, astringent, circulatory stimulant, cognitive support,
neuroprotective, peripheral vasodilator.

Dosage
A daily cup is health rewarding – with break periods of a week or two
every few months. Therapeutic doses in the range of 2–3 daily cups for
duration of treatment.

Caution
Ginkgo is not advised if you are on anticoagulant or antiplatelet medication. It can interfere with MAOI and with selective serotonin reuptake
inhibitor (SRRI) medicines. Recurrent use or overuse can cause some
photosensitivity, gastrointestinal upset or dizziness in some.

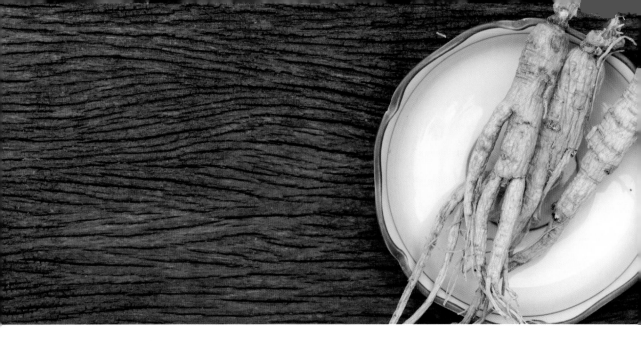

Ginseng Tea

*(Panax quinquefolius, P. ginseng
and Eleutherococcus senticosus)*

Botanical family
Araliaceae

Parts used
Roots

Flavour profile
Earthy to bitter

There are three main types of ginseng readily available: American (*Panax quinquefolius*), Asian, aka Korean or Chinese (*Panax ginseng*), and Siberian (*Eleutherococcus senticosus*). All contain potent health-boosting properties. While in herbalism there may be subtle variances in usage, the types are also considered interchangeable.

How to make
The root is traditionally decocted by simmering the diced fresh or chopped dried root at a ratio of 1–2 teaspoons per cup for 7–15 minutes. Teabag versions can be infused for 3–5 minutes. Ginseng tea can also be served as iced tea.

Health benefits
A treasure of traditional Chinese herbalism, ginseng is employed as a general pick-me-up tonic to remedy fatigue and general debility, and to sustain immune response and convalescence. In Western traditions it is utilised to address adrenal fatigue, chronic fatigue, high blood sugar, high cholesterol, IBS, insomnia, stress and depression, improve

memory and concentration, and slow the progression of dementia and cognitive decline. Being oestrogenic, it also can be used to relieve the symptoms of menopause. Below is more specific detail on the three types of ginseng.

American ginseng is utilised globally as an adaptogenic herb – i.e. to protect against stress of all types (physical, emotional, environmental), to improve physical strength and stamina, and to increase overall wellness. It is also currently under study as a nootropic (intelligence) and cognitive function booster, in particular with working memory enhancement.

Asian ginseng is considered a longevity tonic. It is globally availed of as an energiser to improve mental and physical stamina. It supplies sesquiterpenes – plant chemicals that are beneficial to the prevention of neurodegeneration. It is also beneficial to the relief of pain, inflammation and stress.

Siberian ginseng has a strong reputation as an invigorating tonic and is utilised as a physical and mental energiser and a stress buster. It has been used since the 1960s within the Russian space programme to help cosmonauts acclimatise to space travel/dwelling and to endure the stresses of training. It shares attributes with the other ginsengs.

Main medicinal actions: Adaptogen, analgesic, antidepressant, anti-inflammatory, antispasmodic, anxiolytic, cholinergic, digestive, hypo-glycaemic, hypocholesterolaemic, immunostimulant, nootropic, oestrogenic, vasodilator.

Dosage

The standard is a daily cup for a couple of weeks, then a break period. Therapeutically taken for 3–4 weeks at a time, alternating with a 2-week rest period to boost its efficiency on the next cycle. (Some herbalists may prescribe higher doses of 2–3 cups for a specific treatment at a similar or shorter duration.)

Caution

Avoid in pregnancy and with high blood pressure. Note its oestrogenic action in relation to hormone therapies and oestrogen-related conditions.

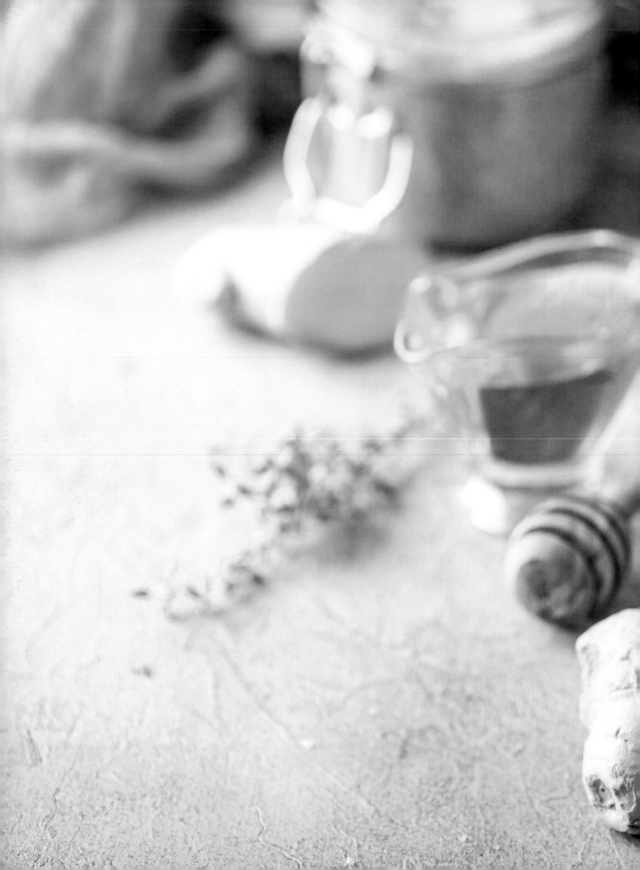

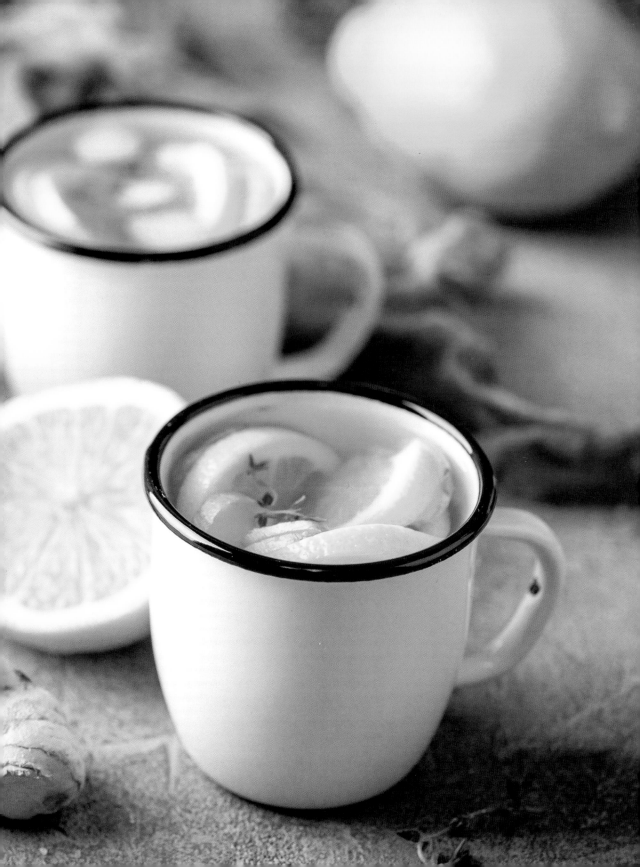

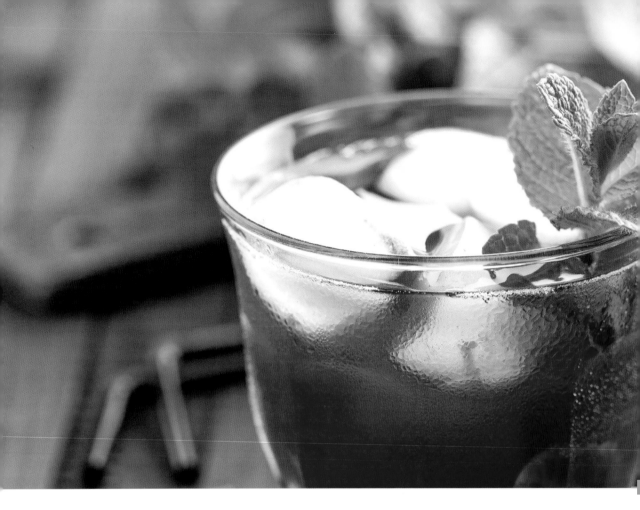

Goji Berry Tea

(Lycium barbarum and *L. chinense)*

Botanical family
Solanaceae

Parts used
Berries

Flavour profile
Tart

Originally Gou Qi Zi, the red goji fruits are traditionally employed in Traditional Chinese Medicine (TCM) to strengthen liver and kidney channels and to nourish blood and Jing (the essence of life) and add potency to male libido and function. You can make a tea from dried berries or find teabag-type 'goji tea' that is generally a blend of the dried berry with white or green tea.

How to make
Older traditions are of a 5-minute simmering decoction. Contemporarily, a tablespoon of dried berries can be hydrated in a cup of boiling water – allow to sit for 5–10 minutes, then the plumped-up berries can be eaten

rather than discarded and thus add some of their additional non water-soluble ingredients to the system. Otherwise drain and sweeten to taste.

Goji have that thing where some berries are tangy with a sweet after-taste and others may be tart. So two cups in the same day may have a slightly different nuance. A dot of honey or stevia takes the sour edge off.

Health benefits

Goji have all the antioxidant punch of 'superfoods' and so have a well-earned reputation as a restorative and anti-ageing herb. They are packed with a set of particularly potent plant chemicals known as proteoglycans and referred to as *Lycium barbarum* polysaccharides (LBPs), which have been studied for their positive pharmacological effects on age-related illness, neurodegenerative complaints and conditions such as atherosclerosis, macular degeneration, glaucoma and diabetes. LBPs support improved blood flow and arterial cleansing, and regulate efficient glucose metabolism.

Goji tea is a brilliant detox. It contains ample betaine – an amino acid which actively reduces fatty deposits in the liver. Betaine also promotes protein synthesis in the body, is involved in both muscle gain and fat loss, and has connections to increased physical performance/endurance. In TCM, goji berry is lauded to enhance both male fertility and sexual performance – the energising betaine and those LBPs validate that somewhat.

Main medicinal actions: Adaptive, anti-inflammatory, antioxidant, anti-viral, cardioprotective, circulatory tonic, hypoglycaemic, hypolipidae-mic, immunostimulant, probiotic, sexual system tonic.

Dosage

1–3 cups daily for specific treatment duration is within the therapeutic range.

Caution

Avoid if allergic to plants in the nightshade family. May interact with blood-thinning medications and potentially in higher doses affect how quickly the liver breaks down other prescription medications. Not advised for use with a spleen deficiency.

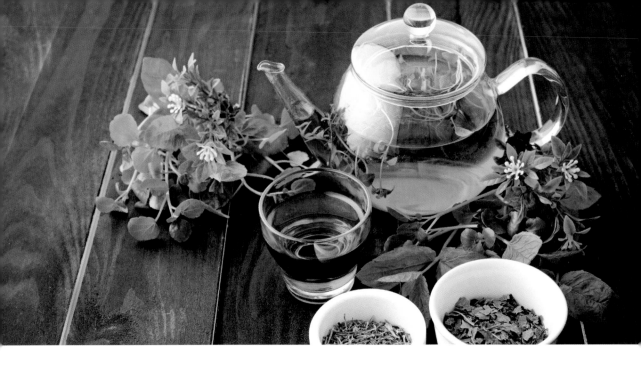

Green Tea

(Camellia sinensis)

Botanical family
Theaceae

Parts used
Budding tips and leaves

Flavour profile
Mild tannin to sweet vegetal

Green tea gets its name from the colour it diffuses upon infusion. There are many varieties of green tea but all are dried at harvest to prevent fermentation/oxidation. It does contain caffeine and is not strictly 'herbal', but increasingly green tea is being mixed with various herbs to create herbal green blends, or stacked alongside herbal teas in the supermarket aisles.

How to make
Green tea was used for the original tea ceremony, so to say that there is a tradition in it is an understatement. Whisking bowl aside, the majority of green tea consumed on the planet is taken in a hot infusion of boiled water which has been allowed a moment to cool below boiling point. Boiling water can make tea more astringent and evaporate off some of the healing phytochemistry. Make in a covered cup or teapot. Infusion rates are traditionally within 1–3 minutes.

Traditionally Chinese green teas are infused at higher temperatures – on average 75–80°C (170–180°F), while Japanese green teas are infused at lower temperatures in the region of 70–75°C (160–170°F).

Differing blends and brands offer variances in flavour – longer brewing can increase bitterness.

Health benefits

Pure green tea is most popularly utilised as a pick-me-up beverage, to restore physical energy and improve mental alertness. Its content helps to support cognitive function and strengthen mental performance via improved cerebral blood flow, and that has a knock-on effect on positive mood/outlook. It also exerts neuroprotective effects.

Green tea is the dominant drive in all blends, no matter what herb it may be mixed with. It brings with it the polyphenol known as epigallocatechin gallate (EGCG) – a potent antioxidant and inhibitor of tumour necrosis factor alpha (a cell-signalling chemical involved in both cancer development and systemic inflammation). This tea is also well known for its chemoprevention of various cancers, including gastric, colorectal, prostate, breast, cervical, pancreatic, liver, lung, oesophageal osteosarcoma and leukaemia. It is also a contributor to weight loss and improved athletic endurance. The EGCG content helps reduce blood levels of ghrelin – 'the hunger hormone' – while increasing levels of adiponectin – a substance active in the breakdown of fatty acids and regulation of how fat is stored or burned.

The various added herbs and flavourings – lemon, mint, lotus flower, jasmine, etc. – will add their own medicinal actions to the pot.

Main medicinal actions: Antibacterial, anticarcinogenic, antihypertensive, anti-inflammatory, antioxidant, antiproliferative, antiviral, cardiotonic, cerebroprotective, chemopreventive, diabetic support, diuretic, neuroprotective, pick-me-up, stress relief, weight loss.

Dosage

The various green tea types vary in their caffeine content but, in general, it is not advised to go beyond 4–5 cups per day so as to avoid caffeine side effects, yet some therapeutic doses do exceed this amount.

Caution

Usual cautions apply with caffeine. The tannin content can increase stomach acidity and interrupt iron absorption.

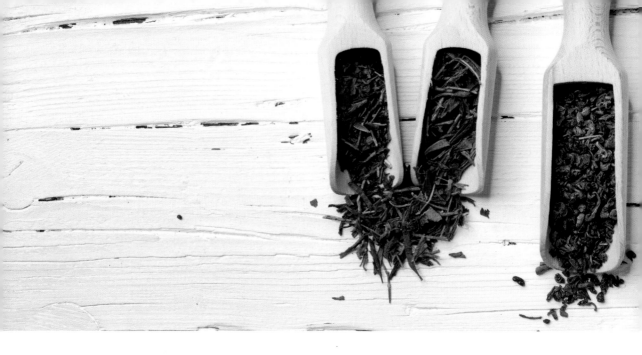

Green Tea Types

Green tea's origin myth is linked to its medicinal and stimulant value long utilised in Asian medicinal systems. Today it is considered to be pharmacologically active against cognitive dysfunction and potentially slows the progression of dementia. The folk use of tea for centuries as a restorer of physical energy and mental clarity, as well as a remedy against stress and emotional shock, is now borne out by what we know of the science of its constituents.

There are many different types of green tea, with nuances in flavour and colour, which are down to growing location and even the microclimate within that location, and the other ingredients with which the leaves are blended – grains, flowers, other herbs. Here are some of the most popular, and while they are notably Chinese and Japanese varieties (my personal preference), other tea-growing regions also produce variances in green tea styles and flavour profile.

Genmaicha is a blend of Japanese steamed green tea (generally a sencha type) mixed with roasted brown rice, aka genmai, which adds sweet, nutty and roasted notes to the flavour. The pleasantness of the flavour may help the health benefits of the green tea content kick in more quickly, as the soothing aroma and taste receptor responses also help lessen tension and anxiety, and step the brainwaves down towards a more relaxed state. The theanine content follows up on the aroma and further alters brain chemistry towards relaxation and positivity perception.

Filled with blood pressure-lowering catechins and all the health benefits of typical green tea, the addition of the roasted rice adds gamma-oryzanol – a substance supportive of pancreas cells and insulin sensitivity. Brown rice contains GABA, a substance that triggers our natural sedation and anti-stress chemistry but which also plays a role in slowing the progression of obesity and diabetic-related complications.

Gunpowder tea is a green tea from China that attained its name via the process of being rolled into small round pellets like grains of gunpowder. These grains don't explode, but they do open up upon infusion and release not just a smoky flavour and aroma but the full array of green tea chemistry, including anti-inflammatory catechins and chemoprotective antioxidants.

Gunpowder tea also contains good quantities of magnesium and fluoride, explaining some of its traditional reputation for oral health and for muscle aches. It is often considered more than a pick-me-up and has gained both reputation and popular usage as an endurance tonic and clarity beverage, perhaps due to its higher levels of caffeine than that found in other green teas – roughly 35–40mg/8oz per serving.

Houjicha is a relatively modern tea, originating in Japan in the 1920s. *Houjiru* is a verb meaning 'to roast' and this is a roasted tea, most often comprised of the leaves of summer and harvests of a later flush. The roasting adds a smoky to nutty to caramel flavour depending on the process. Initially the tea was pan-fried or roasted in a porcelain pot over charcoal; many blends are now roasted in drums similar to the coffee roasting process. The roasting was a break from the older tradition of steaming tea.

The roasting process not only adds nuances to the flavour and body of the tea, but it reduces the caffeine levels, making Houjicha green teas closer to a herbal infusion while maintaining the phytochemistry of green tea.

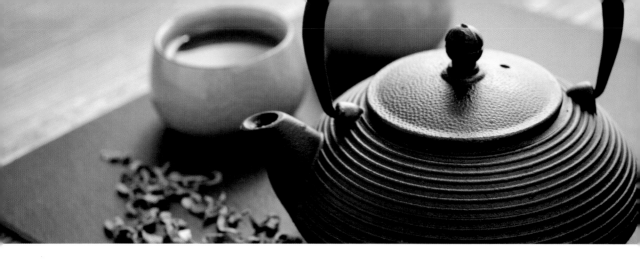

Longjing aka **Dragonwell tea** is a spring harvested Chinese tea, mainly from the Xi Hu district of Hangzhou in the Zhejiang Province. The spring harvest is of young buds primed with antioxidants, and the location's microclimate and soil make it a more chlorophyll-rich leaf and so sweeter to the taste. It is folded into a flat leaf stick before being stabilised via pan-frying. It is a green tea that retains some of its jade colour and higher concentrations of catechins than other types. It was, for most of its history, the tea of emperors. The caffeine content in longjing is lower than in other types but still enough to enhance cognitive acuity and physical endurance – just what every emperor needs.

Matcha translates as 'rubbed tea'. It was traditionally a superior grade of green tea that was stone ground to a fine powder and whisked in a bowl rather than being infused. It could be whisked to usucha (thin tea) or served as koicha (thick tea). The technique of grinding and the whisking with hot water rather than infusing meant one imbibed/consumed more of the tea particles and so more flavour and phytochemicals. This is not the only reason that consuming a cup of matcha delivers roughly as many antioxidants as drinking ten cups of regular black or green tea! Matcha is also grown in the shade and this enriches phytochemical build-up within the foliage.

Matcha is seen as a higher potency green tea. It is quite high in L-theanine, which switches the brain and nervous system to more relaxed states. It entered Japan *circa* AD 1200 via Myōan Eisai, a Japanese Buddhist monk who, while studying in China, noticed how many Buddhist monks drank it to aid their meditation and how its medicinal values were valued outside the monastery too. Eisai eventually returned to Japan and wrote a book called *Kissa Yojoki* all about the benefits of green tea. Its first line is quoted at the beginning of this book. Most matcha tea brands still come in powdered form, but it is also becoming popular in multi-blends and has even sneaked into teabag form.

Sencha translates as 'infused tea'. It became popular in the eighteenth century as an accessible form of tea without the requirement of the traditional tea-whisking technique required with matcha and other green teas. This opened the brew to the masses and allowed its use to step outside of the reverential/ceremonial and into a daily cuppa. It is further differentiated from matcha and gyokuro types by being cultivated in full sunlight (with the exception of the sub-category known as Kabuse sencha). The leaves are stemmed upon harvest to prevent oxidation. Varieties in length of steaming, time of harvest and regional soil variances all deliver nuances in flavour.

Approximately 80 per cent of the green tea processed in Japan is a sencha type – and, yes, there is more than one. Top choices include Shincha ('new tea'), a sweeter, spring season harvest; fukamushi sencha, a stronger tea from second flushes that is often brewed for longer; and asamushi sencha, a variety only lightly steamed to maintain its mild flavour. Chumushi sencha is really a blend of fukamushi and asamushi designed to deliver a mid-strength tea with a slight buttery flavour note. Kabuse sencha is a tea acquired via the cultivation technique of *kabusu* (to cover) – it involves shading the crop during a period of growth in order to encourage the plant to produce more chlorophyll-rich, and so more tender and sweeter, leaves.

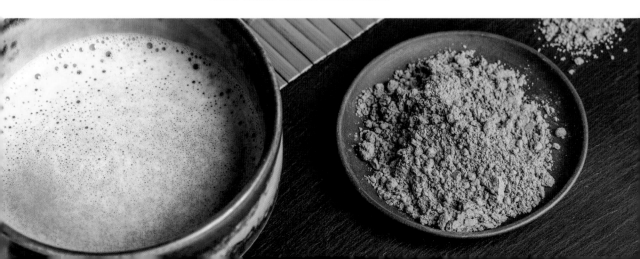

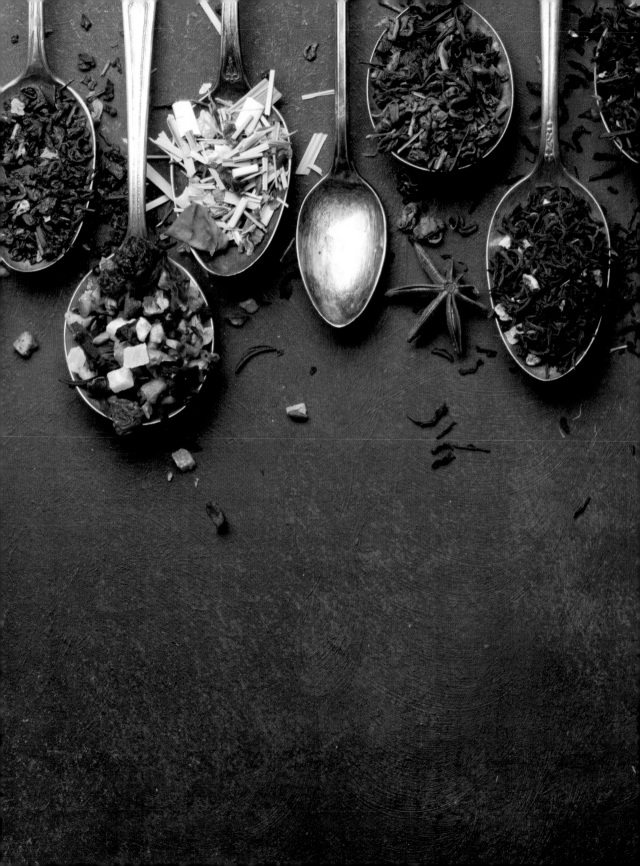

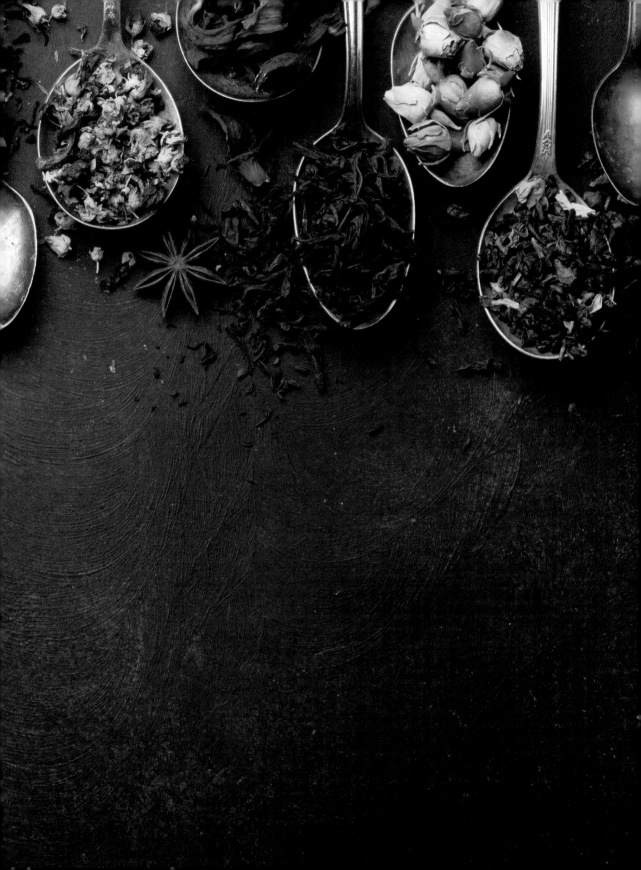

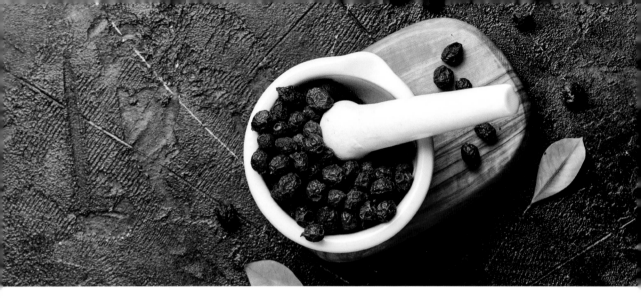

Hawthorn Tea

(*Crataegus monogyna* and *C. oxycantha*)

Botanical family
Rosaceae

Parts used
Leaves, flowers and berries

Flavour profile
Bitter

Traditionally across Europe and where it grows, the leaves, berries and flowers of hawthorn are used to make a range of herbal medicines. The haw in the name derives from the Old English word 'haga', denoting a 'hedge'. The genus name *Crataegus* derives from the Greek *kratos*, denoting strength, and it does make both a sturdy hedge and strong medicine. Proprietary blends of hawthorn tea may be pure leaf or a mix of components.

How to make
Traditionally made by a decoction of plant parts simmered for 10–15 minutes, but a 5–7-minute infusion is as effective in the extraction of phytochemicals. One teabag or 1–2 teaspoons of dried herbage per cup is required, utilising freshly boiled or momentarily rested boiled water. Longer infusions/decoctions can bring out some bitterness, but can be sweetened with stevia or honey.

Pure 'berry tea' (made of the dried berries) is best made via the simmering method.

Health benefits
Hawthorn is a supreme venous and coronary tonic, utilised in the treatment and prevention of a range of circulatory and cardiovascular

disorders: angina, atherosclerosis, arrhythmias, congestive heart failure, hypertension, tachycardia and valvular insufficiency including varicose veins. It is packed with antioxidants that keep the system protected from oxidative stress – a bodily occurrence where the production of free radicals outnumbers our body's ability to counteract or detoxify their harmful effects. Hawthorn also contains phytoconstituents that dilate and tone the smooth muscles of the heart and blood vessels. Its phytochemical content of apigenin, kaempferol, quercetin, luteolin and rutin not only improves the integrity of blood vessels and capillaries, but bolsters general health.

Plant parts contain oligomeric properties that help to strengthen capillaries and tone venous health, and also act to reduce lipid per-oxidation, lower cholesterol levels, reduce inflammation and oedema, and boost the effectiveness of vitamin C and other antioxidants inges-ted from food. It can also slow glucose absorption into the bloodstream and is of benefit in regulating diabetic blood-sugar spikes.

Hawthorn inhibits angiotensin – a peptide hormone which, in excess, increases blood pressure, water retention and levels of potassium and sodium within the system. Angiotensin's main action is in the constriction of blood vessels. The impact upon improved circulation and cardiac function often induces a sense of being energised, and so hawthorn tea has an application in convalescence from illness and also with fatigue and depression. The better supply of blood can improve cognitive function and wellness perception.

Main medicinal actions: Adaptogen, anti-arrhythmic, antioxidant, anti-spasmodic, cardiotonic, coronary vasodilator, hypotensive, nervine, peripheral vasodilator.

Dosage
2–3 cups daily.

Caution
Generally regarded as safe but do check against the contraindications of your current medications as it may increase the potency of some prescription and over-the-counter medications.

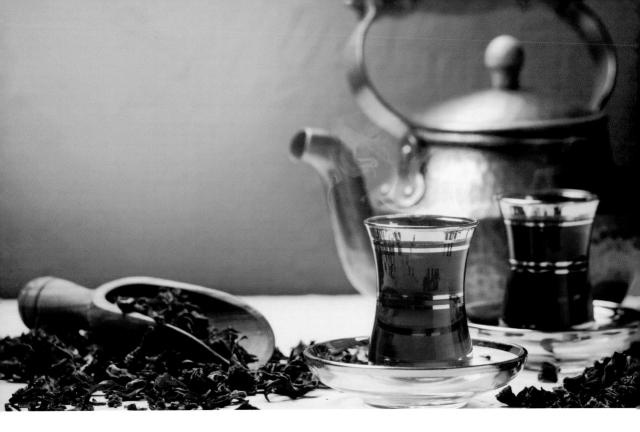

Hibiscus Tea

(*Hibiscus sabdariffa*)

Botanical family
Malvaceae

Parts used
Flowers/sepals

Flavour profile
Sour

While *Hibiscus rosa-sinensis* features in herbalism with many of the attributes listed here, it is *Hibiscus sabdariffa*, commonly known as 'Roselle', that supplies the hibiscus flowers that make the globally popular tea. Sometimes the tea is referred to as 'roselle tea' to distinguish it from the other over 200 species of hibiscus.

How to make
The traditional method of a 'soft decoction' is akin to modern infusion – it involves boiling water in a lidded saucepan, adding two whole hibiscus blossoms or about 2 teaspoons of dried flower petals per cup and resting off the heat for 15–20 minutes. Some versions then simmer a while with plenty of sugar to sweeten the inherent sourness (cranberry-like), but that undermines many of the medicinal benefits. Teabag versions can be infused for 2–7 minutes. Often served at room temperature or chilled as an iced tea.

Health benefits

Its oldest usage includes remedying loss of appetite, treating flu, colds and catarrh, and as a diuretic. Hibiscus flowers are high in vitamin C (20 times higher than an orange) and other antioxidant constituents that benefit well-being as well as illness recovery. It is increasingly being utilised in modern herbalism to help lower blood pressure and remedy conditions with a venous or circulatory connection. Its hypoglycaemic properties are also active in lowering triglycerides and low-density lipoprotein cholesterol, making it a valuable natural co-therapy in diabetes management.

The tea is also utilised as a nervine (to calm the nerves) and as an antispasmodic – making it beneficial in addressing conditions from restless leg to menstrual cramps, but also in the alleviation of migraines and IBS. A strong tea, made from doubling the herb rather than lengthening the steepage time, has value as a laxative and a history in detox treatments, which led to its use as a weight-loss tea. Its success in weight loss is down to its content of an amylase enzyme that breaks down carbs and complex sugars more efficiently.

In some Ayurvedic and Unani texts, hibiscus has a reputation as being antifertility or contraceptive; this may be down to phytoestrogens having a slight antispermatogenic effect in men and by triggering oestrogen fluxes that exert an anti-implantation effect in women.

Main medicinal actions: Anti-oestrogenic, antioxidant, antiviral, appetite stimulant, diuretic, detox, expectorant, hypolipidaemic, hypoglycaemic, hypotensive, laxative, vasodilator, vasoprotective, weight management.

Dosage

Single cup daily to upper range of 2–3 cups for treatment duration.

Caution

May increase the effectiveness of diabetic and blood-pressure medication and lessen the effectiveness of contraception and hormone replacement therapy (HRT) medication.

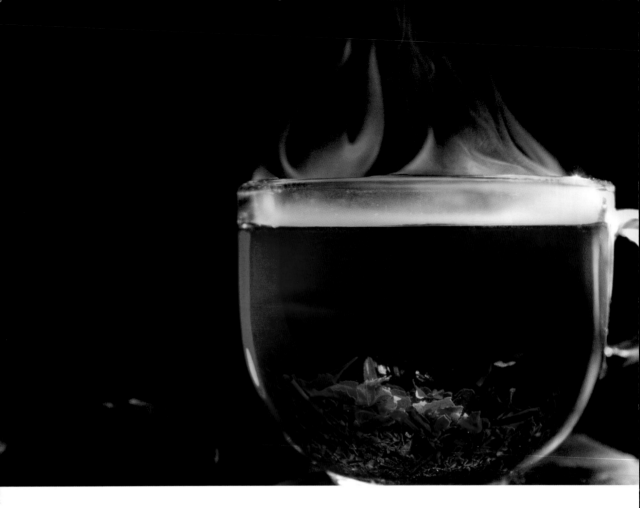

Honeybush Tea

(Cyclopia intermedia)

Botanical family
Fabaceae

Parts used
Leaves, stems and flowers

Flavour profile
Sweet, tangy

A honey-scented, broom-like plant from the pea family that is indigenous to South Africa and is often selected as a tea substitute. Traditionally it is harvested, threshed and left in the sun to oxidise and dry. Modern practices process the foliage over a few days at temperatures of 70–90°C. The result of either method is a tangy tea with no caffeine and lower tannins than black tea.

While *Cyclopia intermedia* is the predominant cultivation, there are regional variations denoting their growing location around the Cape, such as coastal tea (*C. genistoides*), valley tea (*C. subternata*) and Heidelberg tea (*C. sessiliflora*), all with the rich array of antioxidants and phytochemicals that provide the tea's health benefits.

How to make

The tradition is 1–2 teaspoons (to suit personal taste) to be infused in boiling water for a duration of 7–10 minutes or simmered for up to 10–20 minutes. Honeybush tea does not turn bitter with longer steeping or simmering. The resulting tea is often drunk with milk and sugar, in a mimic of black tea, but it can be drunk unadulterated as a herbal tea (better to extract its benefits). It can be served hot or iced.

Health benefits

Honeybush tea is very rich in minerals and some interesting phytochemicals. It contains mangiferin – a major phenolic constituent otherwise found in mangos – which is known to exert antioxidant, anti-diabetic and anti-atherosclerotic actions. The plant yields constituents that offer photoprotection (reduced risk of sunburn) and the tea, both drunk and topically applied (once cooled), has form in remedying the effects of sunburn such as redness, swelling and peeling of the skin.

The plant is a source of xanthones: plant pigments with potent antioxidant, anti-inflammatory and gastroprotective actions, first discovered and isolated by German scientists in 1855 researching dysentery. The honeybush, before being a 'tea', was a local remedy for upset stomachs, chest infections, and aches and pains. The tea supplies a decent quantity of manganese, which attenuates the risk/symptoms of acute joint pain, including arthritis and osteoporosis. Many of the minerals and phenolic compounds found in the tea help to temper the body's inflammatory response and so help suppress pain-triggering mechanisms within muscular structures, which can be helpful with conditions such as IBS or Crohn's disease.

Main medicinal actions: Anti-atherosclerotic, anti-diabetic, antimicrobial, antioxidant, expectorant, gastroprotective, oestrogenic, photoprotection.

Dosage

As a therapy and 'true tea' replacement, upper limits of 2–4 cups daily.

Caution

Generally regarded as safe but usual cautions apply with phytoestrogens that can act to mimic female hormones.

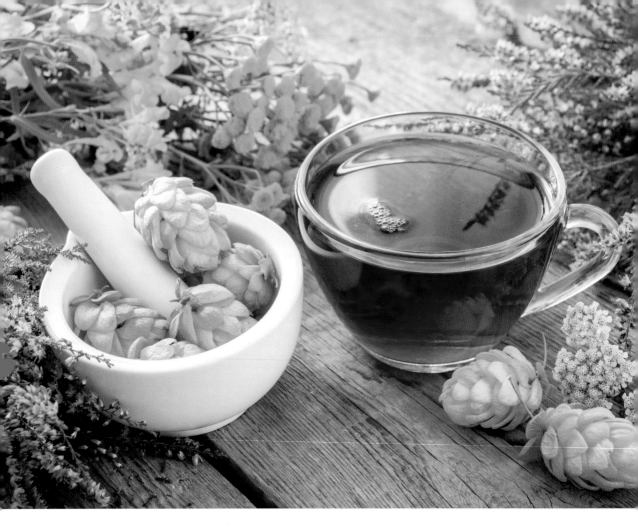

Hop Tea

(Humulus lupulus)

Botanical family
Cannabinaceae

Parts used
Flowering buds

Flavour profile
Bitter

The word hops derives from the Anglo-Saxon word *hoppan*, meaning 'to climb' – a nod to its horticultural habit. Hops have traditionally been utilised to relieve stress and anxiety.

How to make
Hop tea is best produced by a hot water infusion of 10–15-minute duration, traditionally in a lidded teapot with boiling water. The ratio is 1–2 teaspoons of dried herb per cup. Longer steepage can make the taste somewhat more bitter. Teabag blends of hop tea tend to favour a shorter infusion of 4–8 minutes. Both types can be sweetened to taste.

Health benefits

Hypnotic herbs are ones that help with deep and restful sleep and its properties are helpful in addressing hypnotic jerking and restless leg syndrome. The antispasmodic principles of the tea have seen it utilised to quell menstrual pain and also upset stomachs. The oleoresins within the flower heads are bitter substances that will stimulate appetite, gastric secretion and also bile flow, and so have been utilised as a digestive aid as well as a carminative. Constituents within the tea can also address over-colonisation of gut flora by bad bacteria and urinary tract infections.

Hops are packed with phytoestrogens – in particular 8-prenyl-naringenin – which exert in males an anti-androgen effect (aka testosterone blocking). The anti-androgen effect may have potential with testosterone-related issues in women, from both hirsutism and hair loss, to polycystic ovarian syndrome and persistent adult acne. 8-prenylnaringenin also mimics the activity of the female sex hormone oestradiol and can benefit women dealing with menopause and low oestrogen-related symptoms. It can also support female sexual arousal, better vaginal lubrication and more frequent and intense orgasms.

Main medicinal actions: Analgesic, anodyne, anti-androgenic, antibacterial, antiproliferative, antispasmodic, bitter, carminative, chemopreventive, diuretic, galactagogue, hypnotic, nervine, oestro-genic, sedative.

Dosage

Standard use is 1–2 cups daily, generally one in the evening and the other at night for cases of insomnia and other sleep disturbances. Upper limits of 3 cups for other uses.

Caution

8-prenylnaringenin is strong and so not best suited to oestrogen-reactive conditions. Hops can impact upon the efficiency of some contraceptive, antidepressant, insomnia and anxiety medications. It is rare through tea dosages, but excessive consumption of hops can cause dizziness/stupor or next-day drowsiness.

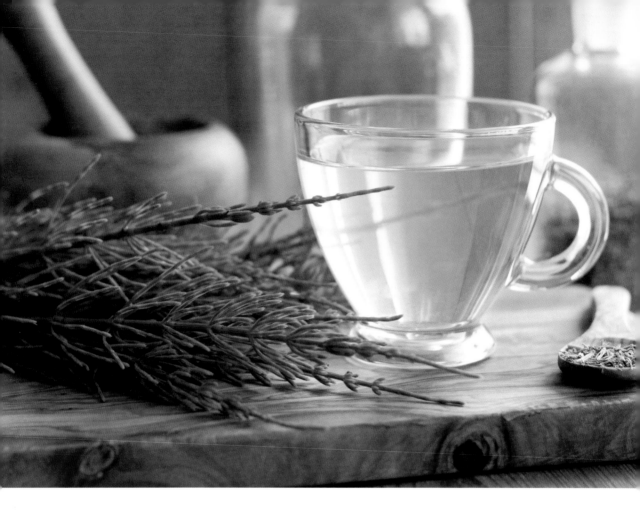

Horsetail Tea

(*Equisetum arvense*)

Botanical family
Equisetaceae

Parts used
Aerial parts

Flavour profile
Herbaceous

The botanical name *Equisetum* derives from the Latin *equus*, meaning 'horse', and *seta*, meaning 'bristle', and denotes how the stem of the plant looks – hence also horsetail as a common name. The silicon content lends it many healing attributes.

How to make
A standard infusion in a cup or teapot with boiling water and a steepage duration of 5–15 minutes. A single teabag or a ratio of 2 teaspoons of dried herb per cup. The taste can be a bit bland; its richer herbaceous notes come out with the longer steepage time. Traditionally sweetened with honey.

Health benefits

Horsetail has a long history as a diuretic to treat prostatitis and urinary tract infections, and to assist in the elimination of kidney and bladder stones. It is also used to address oedema and gout, and in the facilitation of detox routines by helping to eliminate uric acid, lactates and other residual toxins. As a strong diuretic, it can – through prolonged use – cause a loss of potassium and vitamin B1 (thiamin) and so use is often advised against where cardiac or kidney functions may be impaired.

Its astringency and haemostatic properties have seen it utilised to topically treat burns, cuts and wounds. In recent years the silica-rich tea has become popular as a 'beauty tea', being imbibed to rejuvenate the lustre of hair, nails and skin, and also to strengthen connective tissue.

Horsetail helps to increase calcium absorption and can be utilised in prevention and treatment of osteoporosis. Its content can also stimulate immune system activity and be utilised for antioxidant and antiproliferative effects. The tea is also a good source of quercetin, an anti-allergy compound, and is useful prior to flare-up season. If diabetic, the tea also contains the insulinogenic minerals chromium, magnesium and zinc, and the blood glucose-lowering agent beta-sitosterol.

Main medicinal actions: Anti-allergy, anti-atheroma, antihaemorrhagic, anti-inflammatory, antioxidant, anti-rheumatic, astringent, connective tissue tonic, diuretic, genitourinary support, haemostatic, immuno-stimulant, insulinogenic, vulnerary.

Dosage

The upper limit is 2–3 cups daily for short bursts (a week's detox), single cups for longer-term use.

Caution

Not recommended in pregnancy. Horsetail also contains traces of nicotine and other alkaloids that warrant a caution, and a general guidance for therapeutics is restricted to 6-week blocks with break gaps between utilisation: 2 weeks on and 1 week off. This 'blocks and gaps' method is common with many herbs.

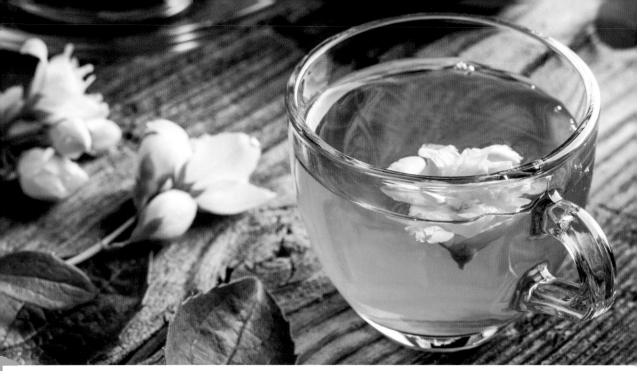

Jasmine Flower Tea

(Jasminum grandiflorum and J. officinale)

Botanical family
Oleaceae

Parts used
Flowers or dried buds

Flavour profile
Sweet, floral

The botanical and common name derives from a French corruption – *jasmin/jessemin* – of the Persian name of the perfumed plant *Yasmin*. There are more than 200 flowering vines in the genus but the most popular are *Jasminum grandiflorum*, which is mostly used in herbal remedies, and *Jasminum officinale*, which is often the preference for aromatherapy, but they are interchangeable.

How to make
Volatile oils contain the main healing actions of jasmine flowers, so boiling water would be too harsh a temperature to extract them intact. Instead, you should allow it to sit off the boil for 30–60 seconds before making a standard infusion. The ratio is generally 1 teaspoon of chopped fresh or dried herbage (flowers) per cup. The infusion should be covered and allowed to steep for 3–6 minutes for best results. Longer brews may taste soapy rather than floral – adjust times to personal taste. Teabag versions are readily available, but read the ingredients to distinguish them from caffeinated, flavoured teas.

Health benefits

Jasmine extracts have been utilised in traditional Indian Ayurvedic medicine to treat gastrointestinal upset, intestinal worms, infections with high fever, viral infection, emotional distress, stress and low libido. In traditional Chinese medicine it is availed of to remedy coughs, sore throats and bronchial ailments, to treat hepatitis and viral infection, and to resolve depression.

Jasmine tea is full of antioxidant flavonoids that not only combat oxidative stress and bolster cellular health, but also help to tone blood vessels, lower blood pressure and help regulate insulin levels. Much of its reputation around its support of weight loss is more appropriately ascribed to green tea flavoured with jasmine.

Jasmine tea is antispasmodic and anodyne in nature, and supports relief from cramping and muscle spasms. When it comes to sedation and mood stabilisation, jasmine's uplifting and soothing aroma has long been employed by aromatherapists to treat anxiety, grief, depression, insomnia, fatigue, anger, libido loss and the whole range of emotional disorders conventionally treated with benzodiazepines, as the aroma activates the same receptors. Properties within the tea also exert anti-inflammatory effects.

The tea has a long-standing reputation for treating female complaints from menstrual issues to breastfeeding to menopause. It is also considered a female aphrodisiac. Topically the cooled tea is utilised to condition skin and hair.

Main medicinal actions: Anodyne, antibacterial, antidepressant, antiseptic, antispasmodic, antiviral, aphrodisiac, astringent, digestive, emmenagogue, emollient, galactagogue, hypotensive, nervine, sedative, thermogenic.

Dosage

Upper limits of 2–3 cups daily as therapeutic dosage.

Caution

Avoid during pregnancy. Note that some of its phytochemistry can have an oestrogenic potential.

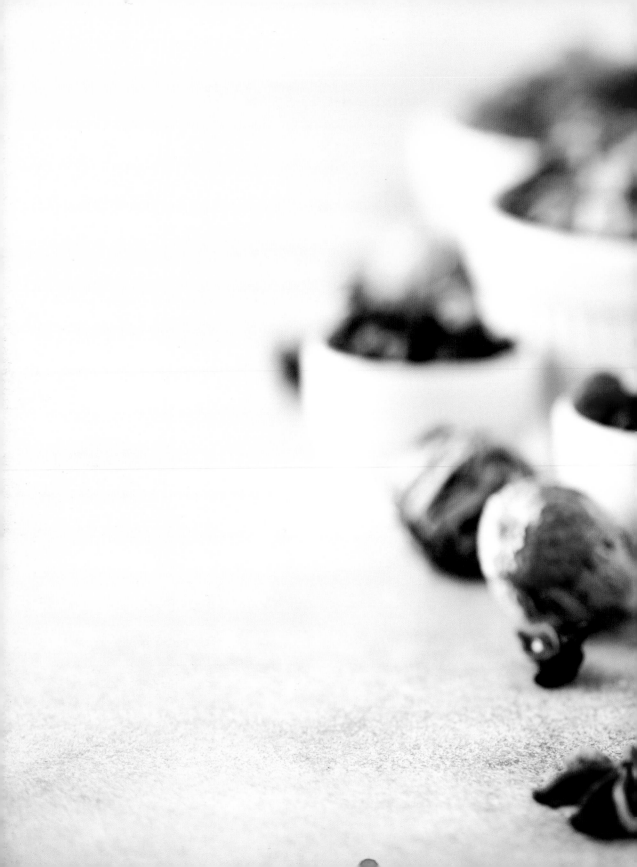

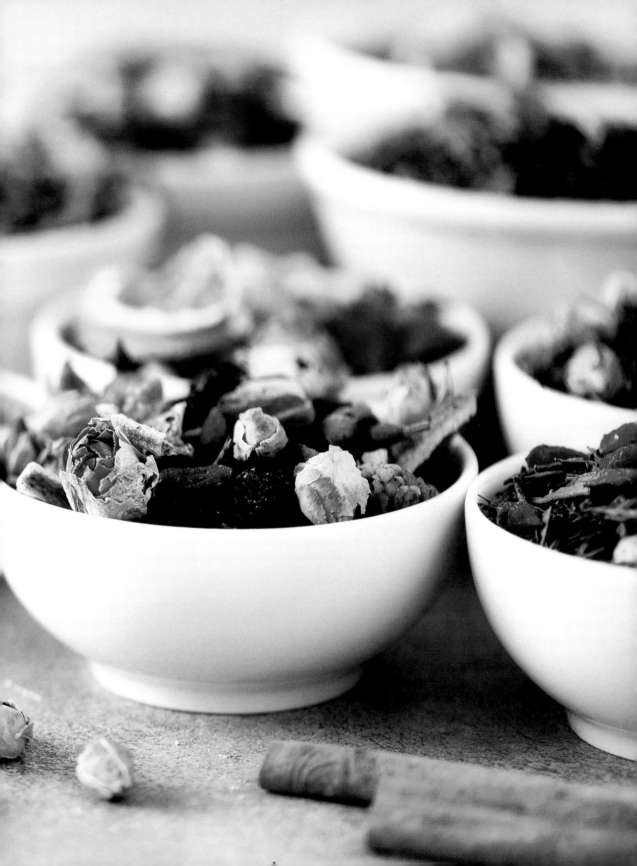

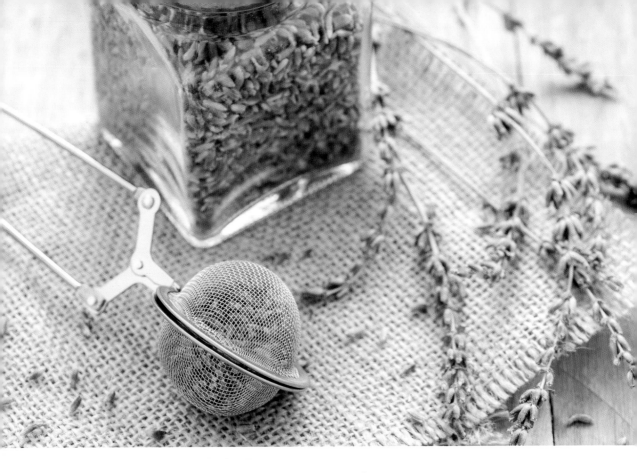

Lavender Tea

(Lavandula officinalis)

Botanical family
Lamiaceae

Parts used
Flowers

Flavour profile
Floral, bitter

There are forty-plus species and hundreds of hybrids all with the same healing potential – so *Lavandula angustifolia*, *intermedia*, *latifolia*, *stoechas*, *vera*, etc., are all good to go. It is listed here as *Lavandula officinalis*, the use of *officinalis* denoting its official status in herbal heritage as an internal remedy.

How to make
As the bulk of its healing potential is via its volatile oils, a covered infusion is best practice. Either a saucer over the cup or a lidded teapot will do. Allow the water to boil, then rest to below boiling point before adding 1 teaspoon of herb (dried or fresh) per cup. I find that the often recommended steepage time of 10 minutes plus can taste a bit soapy, so I suggest you try 3–7 minutes.

Health benefits

The aromatherapy and phytochemistry of lavender is helpful with combating daily stresses, mild depression, generalised anxiety disorder and, according to recent research, with mother/baby bonding and post-partum fatigue. Its volatile oils are recognised as sedative, nervine, anti-inflammatory and antispasmodic. In recent years it has become popular as a remedy for tension headaches, muscular tensions and abdominal cramps associated with both digestive and menstrual issues.

Lauded as a carminative and digestive tea, its antibacterial and antispasmodic nature certainly improves stomach upset, including candida, cramps, abdominal distension and food poisoning. Its cholagogic action promotes the flow of bile and supports healthy digestion. The tea yields blood-thinning coumarins, antioxidant flavonoids and cholesterol-lowering phytosterols that support arterial health. Its potent antioxidant potential is beneficial for cognitive function and mood via enhanced blood flow and nerve and cellular signalling.

Its supply of ursolic acid actively inhibits elastase, a pancreatic enzyme which is implicated in pancreatitis and atherosclerosis, and impacts upon flare-ups of psoriasis and other inflammatory conditions. The cooled tea makes a great skin wash.

Main medicinal actions: Analgesic, antibacterial, anticoagulant, anticonvulsant, antidepressant, antifungal, anti-rheumatic, antispasmodic, antiviral, anxiolytic, carminative, cholagogue, cholinergic, diaphoretic, diuretic, emmenagogue, hypotensive, muscle relaxant, nervous system relaxant, sedative, uterine stimulant.

Dosage

A daily cup is supportive of health; therapeutically the upper limit is 3 cups per day for treatment duration.

Caution

Not recommended in pregnancy due to uterine stimulation. Recurrent or overuse of the tea can cause increased photosensitivity in some. Can potentially interact with conventional anticoagulant and cholesterol medications.

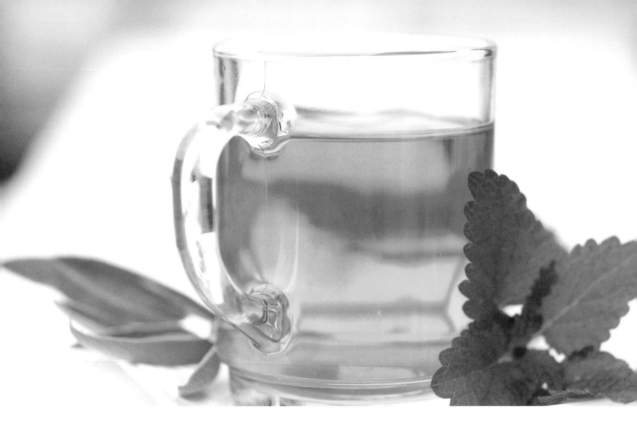

Lemon Balm Tea

(Melissa officinalis)

Botanical family
Lamiaceae

Parts used
Aerial parts

Flavour profile
Lemony

Lemon balm has a long history of medicinal application, stretching back to ancient Greece but peaking in the seventeenth century with a craze for 'Carmelite Water' – brewed by French Carmelite nuns to remedy poor vision, fevers, melancholy, digestive upset and congestion. Today it is popular as a pleasant tea and a remedial beverage.

How to make
1–2 teaspoons of dried herb will match the strength of a teabag. To capture the maximum volatile oils it is best to brew in a pot or cover the cup with a saucer for the duration of the infusion – 3–7 minutes. Fresh leaves can also be utilised and may even taste and smell more strongly of citrus.

Health benefits
The compounds that give it its lemon flavour – citral, citronellal,

citronellol – are antispasmodic agents that work to calm the digestive and nervous systems and are useful in addressing menstrual cramps and tension headaches. The nervine element makes it suitable to remedy IBS and other stress-related illnesses or a stress-related flare-up of underlying illness.

The mood-lifting benefits of lemon balm are delivered firstly through the aroma of a cup and then upon imbibing. Its volatile oils increase acetylcholine levels in the brain – the neurotransmitter with a wide array of tasks, including cognitive function, memory storage and recall, rapid eye movement sleep, as well as neuromuscular signalling and motor control. Significantly, there is often a 70–90 per cent dip in acetylcholine levels in sufferers of Alzheimer's and Parkinson's disease. Cholinesterase inhibitors – which are regularly prescribed to slow the progression of Alzheimer's and Parkinson's – are utilised to prevent the breakdown of acetylcholine by inhibiting the enzymes that destroy the neurochemical. Lemon balm also inhibits those enzymes.

Lemon balm is utilised to tackle anxiety and stress. It contains flavonoids such as apigenin, luteolin, kaempferol and quercetin, which can help improve a general sense of well-being, peripheral blood circulation and cellular health, as well as further supporting acetylcholine levels and action.

Main medicinal actions: Analgesic, antidepressant, antihistamine, antimicrobial, antispasmodic, anti-thyroid, antiviral, anxiolytic, cardio-tonic, carminative, cholagogue, diaphoretic, emmenagogue, febrifuge, hepatic, hypotensive, nervine, nervous system tonic, sedative, stomachic, uterine tonic.

Dosage

A daily cup offers all the actions at safe levels. Do not exceed upper limits of 2–3 cups for specific therapeutics as prolonged use at higher levels may induce a withdrawal sensation for a short period (3–7 days) when treatment ends.

Caution

Avoid with an underactive thyroid.

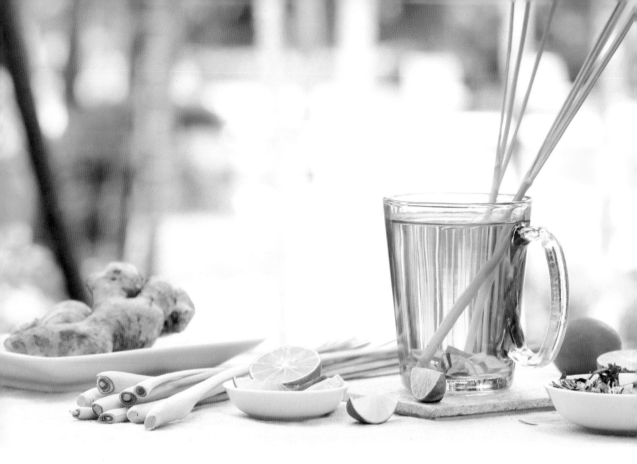

Lemon Grass Tea

(Cymbopogon citratus and *C. flexuosus)*

Botanical family
Poaceae

Parts used
Leaves and stems

Flavour profile
Lemony

Both the common name and scientific epithet – *citratus* – reminds us of its citrus flavour and fragrance. There are around fifty-five species native to Asia and many of those are cultivated around the world. The two most utilised for spice and tea are West-Indian lemon grass (*C. citratus*) and East-Indian lemon grass (*C. flexuosus*).

How to make
Tea can be made from the fresh or dried herb; lemon grass may also be a component of other herbal teas. Older traditions call for a 5-minute boil and an equal length simmer, but I prefer a standard infusion of 3–7 minutes. There are a lot of volatile oils contributing to flavour and taste, so it is best to make it in a teapot or cover the cup with a saucer. Boiling water can destroy some of these healing agents, so let it rest

for 30–40 seconds before applying. Fresh lemon grass can be stronger (acting and tasting) than dried, but ratios tend to remain in the region of 1–2 teaspoons of chopped herbage per cup. Served hot or as iced tea.

Health benefits

Lemon grass is also referred to as 'fevergrass' – a reference to its diaphoretic and febrifuge (fever-reducing) effects. It is also used in Ayurvedic and Chinese medical systems to treat fevers and viral infection. The immune boost of its constituents and its uplifting nature makes it an ideal convalescence tea.

The chemicals responsible for that lemony component are citral, citronellol and limonene, all bearing strong antimicrobial and antifungal properties to quell gastric upset, remedy skin complaints and also to deter insects. Citral in the human system acts as a detox device to stimulate lymph and circulation, and an aid in the removal of fats, toxins and uric acid from the body, making it of benefit to the tackling of arthritis and gout.

Limonene stimulates white blood cell production and inhibits the growth of cancer cells. Citral induces apoptosis (self-destruction) in breast and several haematopoietic cancer cell lines. Citral is oestrogenic and lemon grass tea has a history in treating PMS and menopause. The tea also helps activate the release of serotonin (the happy hormone) and contains a whole plethora of vitamins and minerals conducive to soothing nerve endings and signalling.

Main medicinal actions: Analgesic, anticlastogenic, antidepressant, antifungal, antiproliferative, antitussive, carminative, depurative, detox, diaphoretic, digestive, diuretic, emmenagogue, febrifuge, galacta- gogue, immunostimulant, nervine, oestrogenic.

Dosage

Generally kept within 1–2 cups per day for treatment duration. Iced tea can be sipped throughout the day or at each meal.

Caution

Avoid in pregnancy. May intensify the action of medications for diabetes and anxiety.

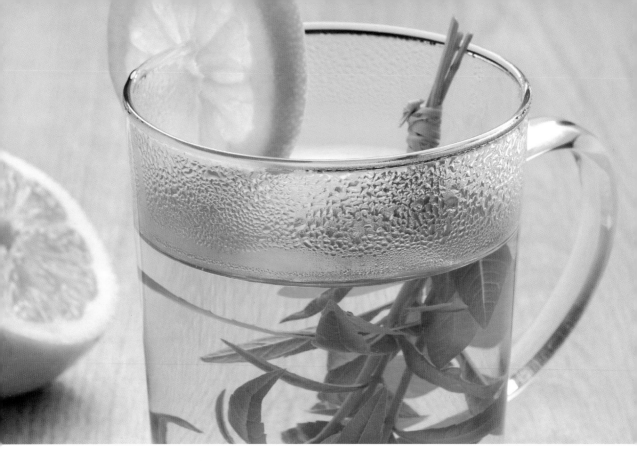

Lemon Verbena Tea

(Lippia citriodora syn. Aloysia triphylla)

Botanical family
Verbenaceae

Parts used
Leaves

Flavour profile
Sweet citrus

In common vernacular 'verbena' denotes a 'leafy branch' and lemon is the fragrance that those branches and foliage emit. *Citriodora* reminds us of that citrus odour. Lemon verbena is a popular tea around the world, often harvested fresh from the garden. It can also be purchased as dried herb or in teabag form. Proprietary blends may include more than pure verbena leaf.

How to make
To preserve the volatile oils that supply its flavour and many medicinal actions, it is best not to use boiling water but allow the boiled water to rest off the boil for 40–60 seconds. Utilise a teapot or cover the cup with a saucer to prevent a speedy evaporation of those components in the rising steam. An infusion in the region of 4–7 minutes is suitable

to yield the full zesty flavour and medicinal potential. 1–2 teaspoons of herbage per cup.

Health benefits

The European tradition with lemon verbena tea is as a citrusy pick-me-up with the benefit of supplying some gastrointestinal action: i.e. in relieving bloating, flatulence, queasiness, stomach cramps and diarrhoea. It also has an application in asthma and bronchial ailments, including tackling excess mucus, coughs and colds.

Many of its constituents, including carvone, dipentene, linalool, limonene, nerol and geraniol, are antiviral and immunomodulating, and it has an application in treating viral infections and also in deterring insects that spread malaria and other viral infections. In South America the tea of this plant is known as 'cedron tea' and its diaphoretic, antipyretic and antispasmodic actions are valued to diminish fever and other symptoms of viral infection.

Lemon verbena essential oil has applications in aromatherapy to alleviate anxiety and depression, and certainly citrus fragrances (and flavour) are energising and uplifting, while the tea's flavonoid constituents work to soothe nerve endings and ease nervous tension, making it a relaxing beverage. The tea's anti-inflammatory nature has some impact on joint pain and it can also help regulate blood pressure and support the efficiency of our immune system, so helps deliver a sense of well-being as well as mitigating illness.

Main medicinal actions: Anti-inflammatory, antimalarial, antipyretic, antiseptic, antispasmodic, diaphoretic, digestive, expectorant, hepatic, hypotensive, nervine, sedative, stomachic.

Dosage

General recommendations are 1 cup over a week to 10-day period, with a break of 3–5 days before restarting in order to limit photosensitivity. In therapeutic doses the upper limit is 3 daily cups for 4 straight days followed by a 3-day break.

Caution

Avoid with kidney complications. Can increase risk of photosensitivity.

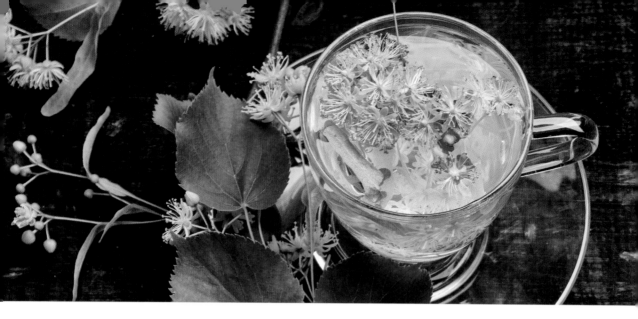

Linden Tea,
aka Lime Blossom Tea

(Tilia cordata and *T. platyphyllos)*

Botanical family
Tiliaceae

Parts used
Flowers

Flavour profile
Sweet

The blossom tea is popular in France as a pleasant beverage and medicinal tea considered to reduce irritability/tension and is utilised for its digestive properties. There are many species, but the traditional lime blossom tea is sourced in the main from either *Tilia cordata* or *Tilia platyphyllos.*

How to make
An infusion is prepared from a teaspoon of flowers per cup. Suffuse in off-the-boil water for 5–10 minutes. Some blends add dried leaf to the mix and this makes a less sweet, more astringent tea. Can be flavoured with honey or lemon.

Health benefits
Linden tea is often thought of as a flu-busting tea, utilised to sweat out the toxins and speed recovery. The vitamin C and other antioxidant and immunity-boosting constituents found in it also help. Furthermore, it has the advantage of reducing and expelling respiratory mucus and

taking the edge off viral and under-the-weather symptoms via its sedative action.

Traditionally serves PMS, insomnia, nervous tension and nervous disorders. As a sedative and hypotensive, it is often employed to alleviate stress and stress-related conditions from fibromyalgia to anxiety to IBS. Over the long term it has proved its worth in addressing high systolic blood pressure, arteriosclerosis and as a co-therapy with degenerative conditions. Circulatory supporting and insulinogenic compounds are also found in the flower.

The plant's properties also deliver a range of beneficial biological activities, including antibacterial, anti-thrombotic, anti-inflammatory, anticarcinogenic and vasodilatory effects. Hesperidin acts on the tonality of blood vessels and may be of benefit to conditions such as haemorrhoids and varicose veins.

Linden also contains beta-sitosterol – a plant sterol ester which is quite similar to cholesterol and, when ingested, helps reduce cholesterol levels by mimicking the presence of cholesterol and thus limiting the amount of cholesterol production within the body. Beta-sitosterol is a component used a lot in conventional medicine to treat enlarged prostates, cervical cancer, psoriasis, fibromyalgia, lupus, arthritis, heart disease and, of course, high cholesterol.

Main medicinal actions: Anticoagulant, anti-inflammatory, anti-spasmodic, anxiolytic, diaphoretic, digestive, diuretic, emollient, expectorant, hypotensive, immunomodulatory, insulinogenic, nervine, peripheral vasodilator, sedative.

Dosage
Standard consumption is 1–2 cups per day. Therapeutic dosages rarely exceed 2–3 cups per day and are confined to low-ish concentrations of herbage and set durations. Generally regarded as safe, but recurrent and higher doses can excite rather than relax the nervous system, causing insomnia, headaches and conditions it is normally set to remedy.

Caution
Avoid in pregnancy or with pre-existing heart conditions (supervision required). Improperly dried blossoms may have narcotic side effects.

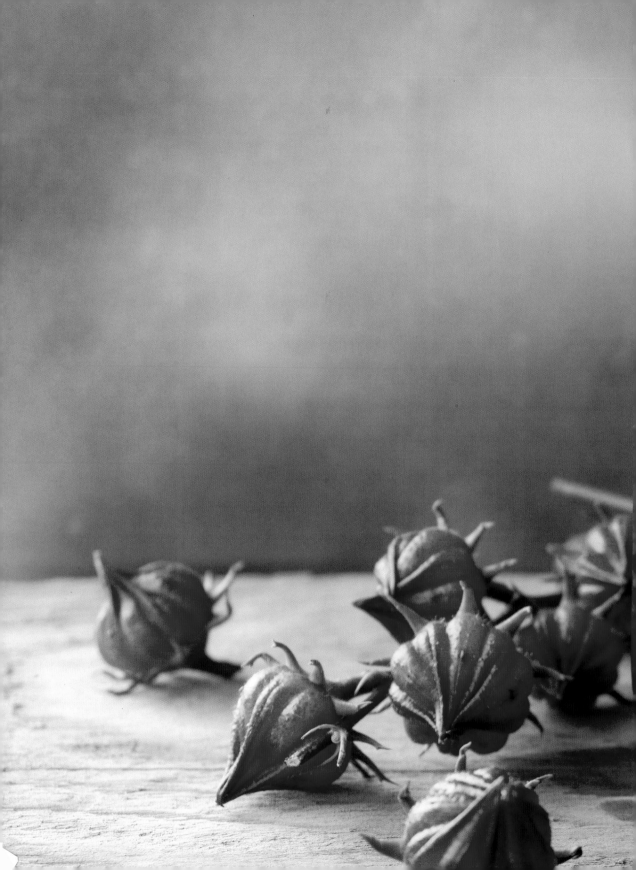

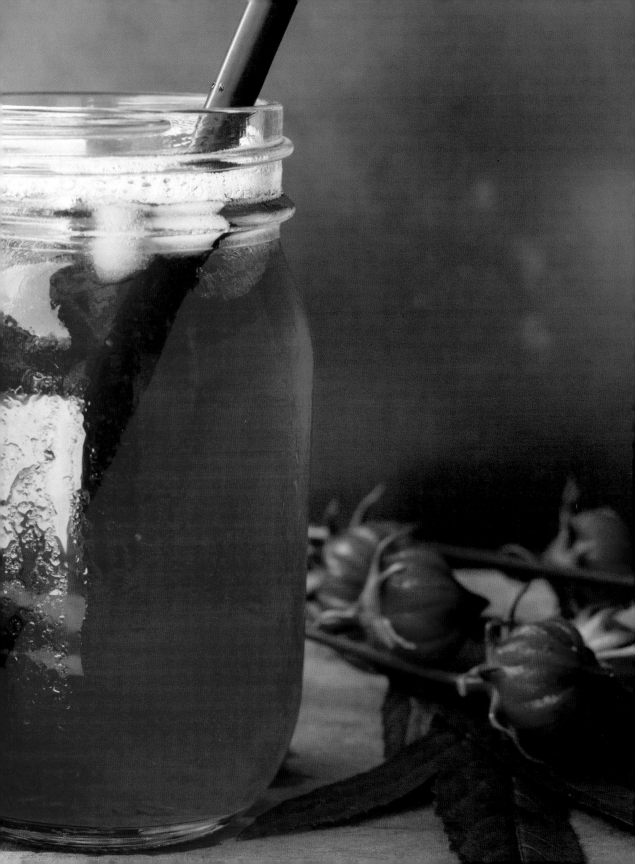

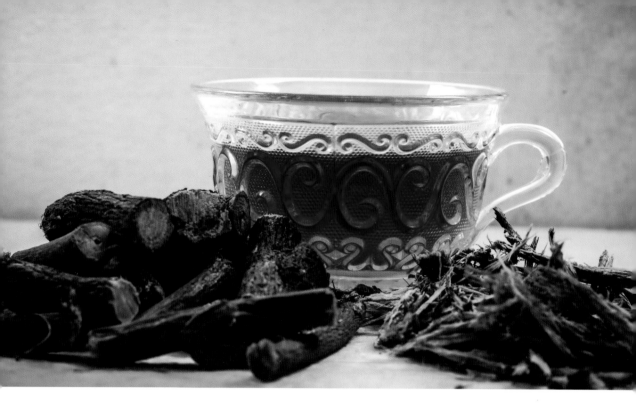

Liquorice Tea

(Glycyrrhiza glabra)

The word liquorice is a corruption of the botanical name 'Glycyrrhiza', which blends the Greek words for sweet (*glykós*) and root (*rhiza*). Liquorice is often utilised in herbal tea blends to enhance flavour.

Botanical family
Fabaceae

Parts used
Roots

Flavour profile
Sweet

How to make
The tradition is via a simmering decoction of 1–2 teaspoons of chopped roots per cup for a duration of 15–20 minutes. Teabags are suited to an infusion with boiling water and a steep time of 4–8 minutes. Liquorice root is sweeter than cane sugar. Can be used as an iced tea.

Health benefits
The triterpene saponins of glycyrrhizin, glycyrrhizic and glycyrrhetinic acid are responsible for liquorice having a very potent oestrogenic action. It also has an application for treating menstrual and menopausal complications, as those saponins also act as natural corticosteroids to lessen inflammation, redness, itching and allergic reactions.

Glycyrrhizin directly modulates enzymes involved in inflammation and attenuates oxidative stress. It may also suppress the growth of certain cancers and tumour cells. Glycyrrhizic and glycyrrhetinic acids exhibit biological activities against liver disease, including the inhibition of hepatic apoptosis and necrosis, and simultaneous promotion of cell regeneration.

Those triterpene saponins are also strongly antiviral in that they both inhibit viral replication and also stimulate an immune system response to viral infection. The plant's rich supply of isoflavonoids are antimicrobial, which means it also has a tradition of use in cold, flu, viral and bacterial infections. It may soon play a role in treatments for Lyme disease and more pernicious infections. Liquorice root is also considered an adaptogen – helping to lessen physical and mental stresses – and beneficial to adrenal insufficiency, chronic fatigue and the stress of long-term illness.

Liquorice tea helps to lower stomach acid and has form in the relief of heartburn and indigestion; it reduces gastrointestinal inflammation and spasm and is sometimes used to treat gastritis, GERD (GORD), IBS and other conditions of the digestive tract. It is also beneficial in soothing sore throats and remedying dry coughs, chest infections and asthma. It has many anti-allergy actions applicable to pollen and histamine reactions.

Main medicinal actions: Adaptogen, adrenal support, adrenocorticomimetic, antacid, anti-inflammatory, antispasmodic, antitumour, antitussive, demulcent, expectorant, hepatoprotective, laxative, oestrogenic.

Dosage
Upper limits of 2–3 cups per day, often with breaks, or a week off week on strategy. In general, unbroken therapies do not exceed six weeks.

Caution
Avoid in pregnancy. Strong oestrogenic action could complicate male fertility. Prolonged use can raise blood pressure, increase sodium retention and reduce thyroid function. Can interact with the efficiency of MAOIs, blood-pressure medications and hormonal therapies.

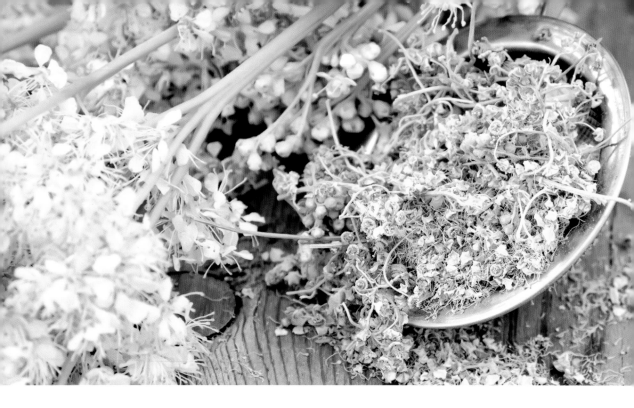

Meadowsweet Tea

(Filipendula ulmaria)

Botanical family
Rosaceae

Parts used
Aerial parts

Flavour profile
Sweet/astringent

Meadowsweet had long been utilised in traditional herbalism to diminish pain perception, ease inflammation and thin blood. In 1897 the German chemist Felix Hoffmann produced a new pain-relief compound – acetylsalicylic acid – later branded as 'aspirin', which was based upon the phytochemistry of meadowsweet. Meadowsweet tea or dried herb may be more readily found in health stores than convenience stores. It can also be garden grown or foraged.

How to make
While the roots have traditionally been utilised in decoction for medicinal application, meadowsweet tea is actually an infusion of aerial parts. The fresh or dried herb is best infused in boiling water for 3–6 minutes at a ratio of 1–2 teaspoons per cup. Longer steepage times will yield a more bitter beverage. Available in teabags and as loose herbage. Some commercial teas may not have the full almond scent of the freshly harvested or home-dried flowers.

Health benefits

The plant chemicals known as salicylates (salicin, salicylic acid) in meadowsweet have seen the herb long employed to treat pain and inflammation. This 'aspirin' effect, combined with its ability to prompt the excretion of uric acid, has great value in remedying arthritis and gout, and in dealing with the pain of other musculoskeletal conditions. Meadowsweet's success with quelling inflammation may also lie in how it attenuates immune response by inhibiting both T-cell proliferation and the production of reactive oxygen species, all of which cools the inflammatory response.

Meadowsweet tea helps to regulate gastric acid levels and actively protects gastrointestinal mucous membranes. It is used as a remedy to treat peptic ulcers, gastritis and heartburn. Like many others in the rose family, it has a traditional usage to remedy diarrhoea and, via its astringency and analgesic principles, to remedy heavy periods. Meadowsweet contains rutin, which can help to strengthen blood vessels and has been utilised in treatments for varicose veins and venous insufficiency.

Plant chemicals within meadowsweet may also be beneficial in alleviating a painful side effect of cancer treatment called mucositis, i.e. swelling and ulcer formation in the mouth that sometimes includes the lining of the digestive tract. Its antimicrobial, astringent and venotonic properties have seen it transition into cosmetic topical treatments.

Main medicinal actions: Analgesic, antacid, anticoagulant, antiemetic, anti-inflammatory, anti-rheumatic, antiseptic, astringent, carminative, diaphoretic, digestive, diuretic, hepatic, mucoprotective, venotonic.

Dosage

Generally a daily cup, but upper limits of 2–3 cups a day in some treatment regimes.

Caution

Avoid if allergic to salicylates or aspirin. Avoid if on blood-thinning medication. Caution with asthma.

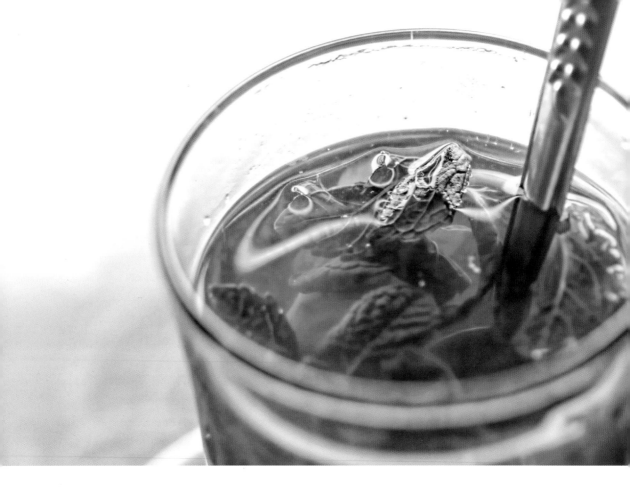

Mint Tea

(Mentha spp)

Botanical family
Lamiaceae

Parts used
Aerial parts

Flavour profile
Menthol

There are many types of mint – *mentha* is a genus of around twenty-five species with hundreds of crosses and cultivars. The two most popular species utilised are peppermint and spearmint, and they have separate entries here so as to cover their medicinal values with some degree of justice.

Some brands of 'mint tea' may be a blend of several varieties and may include specific mints such as garden mint (*Mentha sachalinensis*), Corsican mint (*Mentha requienii*) or Moroccan mint (*Mentha spicata* var. *crispa* 'Moroccan'). Moroccan mint plant in a tea should not be confused with Moroccan mint tea, aka Maghrebi tea, which is a green tea prepared with spearmint and sugar. Some 'mint teas' are green tea blends flavoured with mint.

How to make

Best made by covered infusion to keep the volatile oils from escaping in the steam. The ratio is 1 teaspoon of chopped herbage (fresh or dried) per cup. Use boiled water that has cooled to below boiling for 30 seconds to 1 minute. Allow to infuse for 5–10 minutes. Can be sweetened to taste or flavoured with a little lemon. Pleasant too as an iced tea.

Health benefits

Mint is a superior digestive herb and traditionally utilised to remedy a wide array of gastrointestinal disorders. It is traditionally used to cool the body in times of heat and also stress or agitation. It is further used to remedy dizziness, motion sickness, nausea and headaches. It is beneficial to the respiratory system and helps to alleviate allergy symptoms. The menthol and the rosmarinic acid content of the tea are potently anti-inflammatory.

The antioxidant intensity of mint and its DNA-protecting phenolic compounds have seen mint consumption (and its phytochemicals in scientific isolation) associated with reduced risk of cancer, diabetes, cardiovascular disease and neurodegenerative complications. Topically the cooled down tea helps to cool pain and agitation in muscles and nerves.

Main medicinal actions: Analgesic, antiemetic, anti-inflammatory, antimicrobial, antipruritic, antiseptic, antispasmodic, antitussive, bronchial dilator, carminative, cholagogue, decongestant, diaphoretic, digestive, emmenagogue, nervine, peripheral vasodilator, respiratory support.

Dosage

A daily cup is health boosting. Therapeutic upper limit is 3–4 cups for treatment duration.

Caution

Menthol may inhibit the CYP3A4 enzyme, which is relied upon for the efficient metabolism of some pharmaceutical medications.

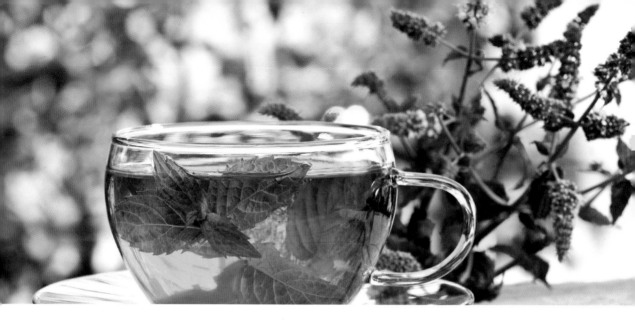

Mint Tea, Peppermint

(Mentha x piperita)

Botanical family
Lamiaceae

Parts used
Aerial parts

Flavour profile
Menthol

Peppermint is actually a hybrid of spearmint (*M. spicata*) and water mint (*M. aquatica*) that occurs naturally in the wild and is also cultivated as a medicinal herb and food flavouring. There are many variations, but the two most recognised and utilised are black peppermint (*Mentha x piperita vulgari*) with darker stems and a reddish flush, and the paler and milder white peppermint (*Mentha x piperita officinalis*).

How to make
A covered infusion traps more volatile oils. Make with water that has been boiled but left to sit until just below boil temperature. The ratio is 1 teaspoon of chopped herbage (fresh or dried) per cup. Allow to infuse for 5–10 minutes. Peppermint has a more intense menthol flavour than other mints but can be sweetened with honey, stevia, lemon, etc. Served hot, or chilled over ice.

Health benefits
Widely utilised as a digestive and carminative to quell stomach upset, gas, dyspepsia and also nausea and motion sickness. Peppermint tea improves the flow of bile and fat digestion. Its antimicrobial action is effective against *Helicobacter pylori*, *Salmonella enteritidis*, *Escherichia*

coli and MRSA, as well as fungal and viral infections. Its antispasmodic potential not only soothes the muscle of the stomach and intestines, but also relaxes the oesophageal sphincter and so helps trapped gas become a burp.

Availed of as a respiratory support, the tea can relieve allergic rhinitis, sinusitis, cold-related stuffiness and seasonal allergies. Its menthol molecules help calm inflamed mucous membranes in the sinuses and actively thin mucus, decongest phlegm and contribute an antitussive effect. It contains several flavonoid glycosides – including eriocitrin, narirutin, hesperidin and luteolin-7-O-rutinoside – that exert an inhibitory effect on histamine release from mast cells, and so quell allergic and inflammatory reactions.

Its rosmarinic acid encourages the production of vasodilating prostacyclins, which consequently inhibits the production of pro-inflammatory chemicals, including leukotrienes, which are the prime triggers of bronchoconstriction in asthmatic attacks. Peppermint also relieves tension and migraine headaches by opening up constricted blood vessels in the brain. The same mechanism may point to benefits in relief from 'brain fog'.

Main medicinal actions: Analgesic, antiemetic, anti-inflammatory, antimicrobial, antipruritic, antiseptic, antispasmodic, antitussive, bronchial dilator, carminative, cholagogue, decongestant, diaphoretic, digestive, emmenagogue, nervine, peripheral vasodilator, respiratory support.

Dosage

A daily cup is health boosting. A single cup can be rationed and sipped at each meal time or a ½ cup half an hour before meals. Therapeutic upper limit is 2–3 cups for treatment duration.

Caution

Avoid with gastro-oesophageal reflux disease and other reflux conditions. May worsen heartburn during pregnancy. Avoid if anaemic. As menthol can inhibit the CYP3A4 enzyme involved in the effectiveness of certain prescription medications, avoid if your meds warn against grapefruit juice.

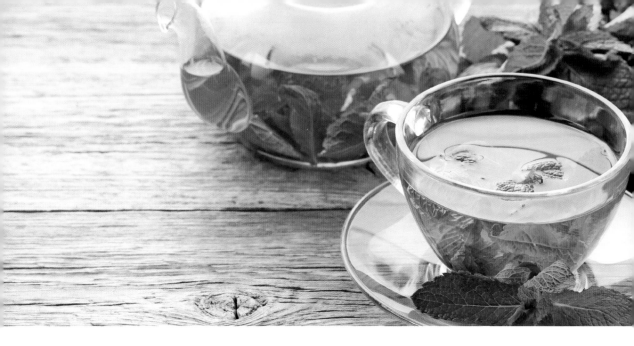

Mint Tea, Spearmint

(Mentha spicata)

Botanical family
Lamiaceae

Parts used:
Aerial parts

Flavour profile
Menthol

Spearmint – sometimes also referred to as garden mint (being popular in cultivation) – is thought to be a corruption of spire-mint and a nod to the pyramidal shape of its flower. The spear-shaped foliage is echoed in *spicata*, a Latin word denoting 'spiked'.

How to make
Spearmint tea can be sourced direct from a garden plant, as a dried herb in a health store, or in teabag form from regular tea stockists and supermarkets. To best preserve the volatile oils, allow boiled water to rest for 1 minute and make in a teapot or cover a cup with a saucer to prevent evaporation during the infusion. The ratio is 1 teaspoon of chopped herbage (fresh or dried) per cup. Allow to infuse for 5–10 minutes. Spearmint is less pungent than some other mints and is pleasant sweetened with honey, stevia, lemon, etc. Can be served hot, or chilled to serve over ice.

Health benefits
Spearmint is often the choice for more tender stomachs; it has less menthol but still delivers digestive, carminative and antispasmodic

action to IBS and Crohn's disease, and is traditionally used to resolve traveller's diarrhoea, food poisoning, sluggish digestion, flatulence, heartburn, indigestion, nausea and travel sickness. Spearmint is also utilised to stimulate liver and gall bladder function and as a remedy for an upset stomach during viral infection, notably the winter vomiting bug.

Spearmint's strong anti-androgenic action can help support the removal of free testosterone from both male and female systems without diminishing what is known as entire testosterone or dehydroepiandrosterone (DHEA), or compromising healthy oestrogen levels. This makes it beneficial in the treatment of benign prostatic hyperplasia and endocrine-related cancers of the prostate in older men. It can also be beneficial in addressing female pattern hair loss and facial hair growth issues in menopause, as excess androgens are often at the root of menstrual irregularities, as well as fertility issues and cystic acne.

Spearmint increases both follicle-stimulating hormone and luteinising hormone, thereby supporting ovarian follicle health, ovulation and regular menstrual cycles. The tea also helps alleviate PCOS-triggered adrenal fatigue and tempers many of the issues contributing to fibromyalgia and other chronic pain/distress syndromes.

Main medicinal actions: Analgesic, anti-androgenic, antiemetic, anti-inflammatory, antimicrobial, antipruritic, antiseptic, antispasmodic, antitussive, bronchial dilator, carminative, cholagogue, decongestant, diaphoretic, digestive, emmenagogue, nervine, peripheral vasodilator, respiratory support.

Dosage

A daily cup is health boosting. Therapeutic upper limit is 3–4 cups for treatment duration.

Caution

Spearmint tea is contraindicated with pregnancy, in incidences of kidney disorders and liver disease. And while less potent in menthol than other mints, it can complicate the efficiency of some enzymes involved in metabolising some prescription medications.

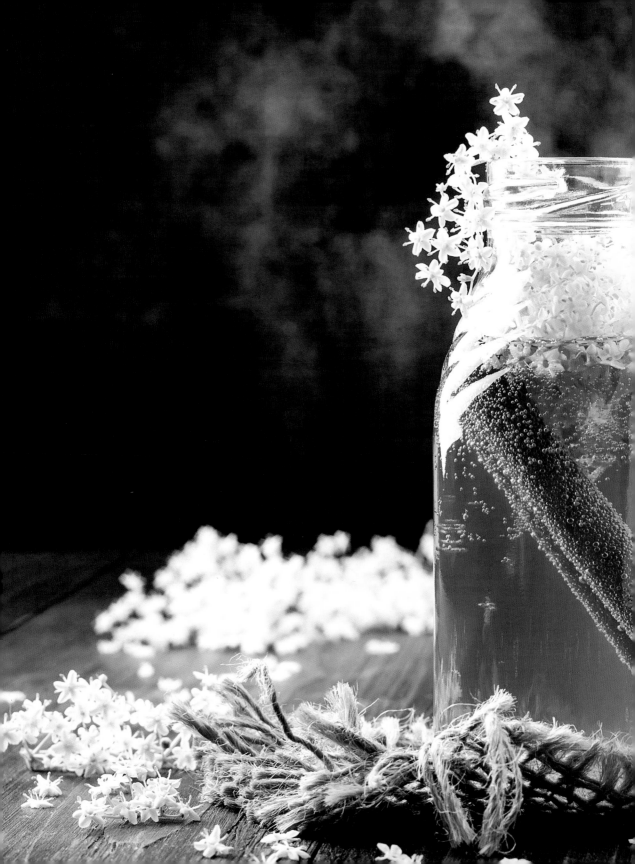

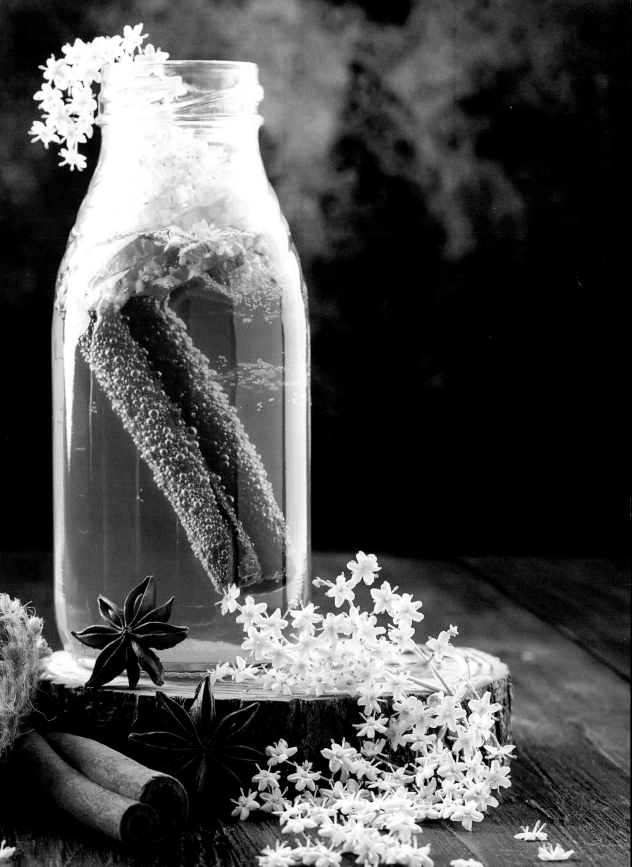

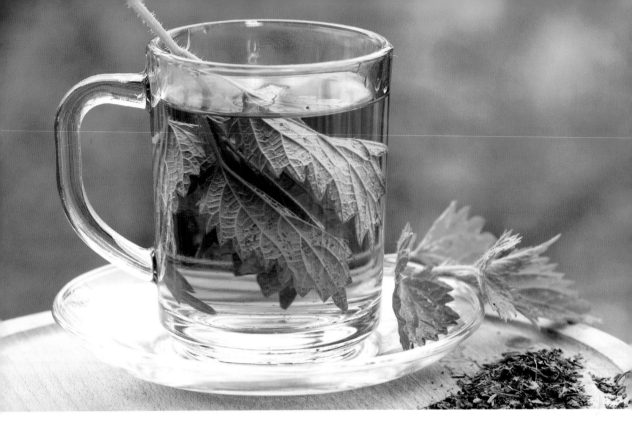

Nettle Leaf Tea

(Urtica dioica and *U. urens)*

Botanical family
Urticaceae

Parts used
Leaves and stems

Flavour profile
Vegetal, bitter

There are two types of nettle commonly utilised in herbalism: perennial or common nettle (*Urtica dioica*) and annual nettle (*Urtica urens*). Both share similar medicinal properties and are used interchangeably. Both also have protective hairs that sting. *Urtica* derives from the Latin *uro* meaning 'to burn'. Heat deactivates the sting.

How to make
Nettle tea can be sourced fresh from the garden, found dried in health stores or in teabag form in the local supermarket. Nettle leaf tea can include the stem, but note that stems hold more bitter principles than the leaves. It is best made by infusion with boiling water and allowed to steep for 5–10 minutes. Depending on the strength required, 1–2 teaspoons of chopped herb per cup. Fresh nettle is much more vegetal in flavour, while dried can lean towards the bitter. Both can be flavoured with lemon or sweetened to taste.

Health benefits

Traditionally utilised as a spring tonic, being rich in iron, silica, potassium, calcium, chromium, magnesium, manganese and zinc, as well as constituents that promote activity of the liver, gall bladder and kidney. Nettle's flavonoids and high vitamin K content make it strongly diuretic and beneficial in the treatment of oedema, cystitis and urethritis, as well as having a long history in prompting the excretion of toxins and uric acid to tackle flare-ups of psoriasis, arthritis and gout.

Nettle tea is seen as a blood tonic and circulatory stimulant. It is also a traditional treatment for anaemia, as the iron and other minerals benefit the production of red corpuscles. It is rich in antioxidants that mop up free radicals and tone the vascular system. It contains medically active compounds such as chlorogenic acid, sterols and glucoquinones that further benefit diabetics, by helping to maintain lower sugar levels and to limit the progression of diabetic neuropathy.

It is an antihistamine via content, which very effectively switches off the production of histamine at its source in mast cells. Other flavonoids found in the nettle leaf, like kaempferol and rutin, are also anti-allergenic and supportive of a healthy and efficient immune system. Nettle impacts upon hormone levels and helps to address symptoms of PMS and menopause, and so may also be beneficial for some prostate disorders in men and for hormonal hair loss in women. Externally, the cooled tea can be used as a hair and scalp tonic.

Main medicinal actions: Anti-allergenic, antihistamine, anti-inflammatory, anti-rheumatic, antiseptic, astringent, circulatory stimulant, detox, diuretic, expectorant, galactagogue, haemostatic, hypoglycaemic, hypotensive, nutritive, tonic, vasodilator.

Dosage

Therapeutic dosage in the range of 1–3 cups a day.

Caution

May increase the actions of diuretics, anticoagulant and antihypertensive medications.

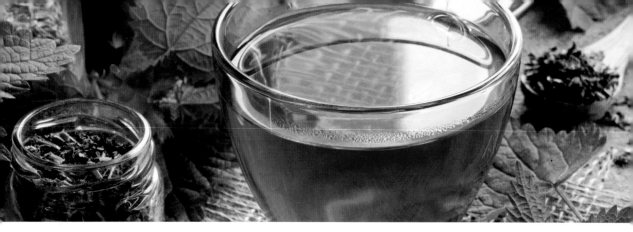

Nettle Root Tea

(Urtica dioica and U. urens)

Botanical family
Urticaceae

Parts used
Roots

Flavour profile
Bitter

Nettle root has many of the same attributes as the aerial parts and has similar herbalism applications. Dried nettle root is generally sold separately as a medicinal herb in health stores, as proprietary 'nettle tea' is generally a foliage and stem tea, but some blends may include all parts. It can be sourced from the garden and oven dried.

How to make
Nettle root tea is best made via a decoction – the cleaned fresh roots or dried root can be brought to a fast boil and then simmered for 5 minutes. I like to let it rest off the heat for a further 3 minutes (just to allow a full leaching of chemicals into the water). Afterwards, strain and sweeten to taste. Longer cooking times can lead to the tea becoming more bitter. The ratio is generally 1–2 teaspoons per cup.

Health benefits
The root is packed with polysaccharides that play a key role in maintaining cellular health, in blood pressure management and in energy metabolism. Antioxidants also found in the tea support general well-being, as well as slowing or inhibiting damage from oxidative stress. Phytochemicals in the nettles also play a role in the suppression of our inflammatory response and have an impact on sex hormones that make this root tea so special.

The roots are packed with plant sterols and steryl glycosides, which one may recognise from cholesterol-lowering yoghurts, but which also have some potent activity in reducing levels of sex hormone-binding globulin (SHBG) protein. The result for men is that it keeps available 'free testosterone' active in the body for longer and continuing to play its role in cognitive function, muscle building and libido. The pathway of reduction of SHBG also inhibits conversion of male hormones to oestrogen metabolites, making it beneficial to the treatment of benign prostatic hyperplasia.

Nettle root tea works to bind to SHBG so that testosterone does not have the opportunity to bind to it. This action dramatically increases the levels of free testosterone available, the kind of testosterone that works positively on the body, the mind, the soul. For women, nettle root works similarly by blocking SHBG. SHBG has an affinity for all sex hormones, and keeping levels of free oestrogen is important in women, just as keeping levels of free testosterone is important in men. For most healthy individuals, high levels of oestrogen and testosterone are damaging only after they have become bound to SHBG, as this begins the process of being converted into harmful oestrogen metabolites, like oestradiol. By keeping these sex hormones free, the rates of conversion to harmful metabolites are decreased.

Excess oestradiol is implicated in hypertension, fibroid develop-ment and growth, endometrial hyperplasia and also with endometrial, ovarian and breast cancers. That said, oestradiol is used in some brands of contraceptive pill and is sometimes prescribed to treat symptoms of menopause, such as hot flushes and vaginal dryness.

Main medicinal actions: Anti-allergenic, anti-androgenic, antihistamine, anti-inflammatory, antiproliferative, anti-rheumatic, circulatory stimu-lant, detox, diuretic, haemostatic, hormonal balance, hypotensive.

Dosage
A daily cup is supportive of health. Therapeutic dosage in the range of 1–3 cups a day.

Caution
May increase the actions of diuretics, anticoagulant and antihyper-tensive medications and interact with contraceptive and hormonal medications.

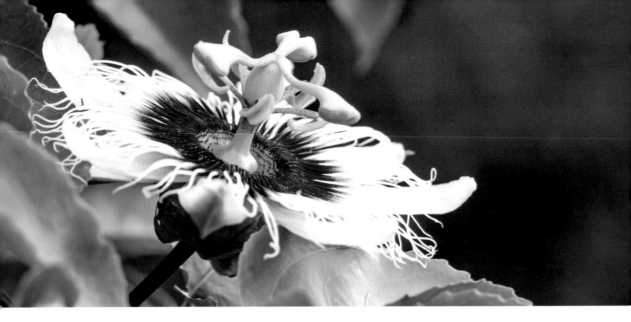

Passionflower Tea

(*Passiflora incarnata*)

Botanical family
Passifloraceae

Parts used
Aerial parts

Flavour profile
Savoury, grassy

The plant has a long ethnobotany tracing back to the Aztecs. *Passiflora incarnata* is utilised in modern herbalism as opposed to the popular garden-grown *Passiflora edulis* (of the edible fruit fame). Generally it is the foliage and stems that are used, but in some proprietary blends the dried flowers may also make an appearance.

How to make
Standard infusion of 3–7 minutes with 1 teaspoon of dried herbage per cup. While passionflower herb doesn't drastically increase in bitterness with longer steepage, the extraction of health molecules is pretty much done after 5 minutes. The tea is pleasant enough but do not expect the fruit flavour. It is suited to some sweetening or flavour enrichment.

Health benefits
Passionflower is a superior calming herb, utilised to settle nerves and quell excessive nerve signalling. It has treatment applications with neuralgia, uterine pain, gastrointestinal spasms, insomnia, irritability and depression. It is having a renaissance in contemporary herbalism to treat generalised anxiety, stress syndromes and opiate withdrawal. It increases levels of GABA within the brain, thereby lowering the

activity of brain cells associated with tension, stress and anxiety. Its array of flavonoids (including rutin, kaempferol, quercetin and vitexin) are antispasmodic, anti-inflammatory, antioxidant, nervine and neuroprotective, while two of its alkaloids (harman and harmaline) exert muscle relaxant and sedative effects, further prompting a deeper relaxed state.

These physical effects upon the body and brain chemistry may relieve chronic pain syndromes, including fibromyalgia and ease conditions such as ME, MS and Parkinson's disease. Passionflower tea has had a history with nervous disorders and their side symptoms of twitches, tremors, headaches, nervous stomach and restlessness, etc. This brew was also once popular in treating 'hysteria'.

Passionflower tea has a good reputation in remedying the symptoms of menopause, including hot flushes, night sweats, confusion and depression. The tea may also benefit erectile dysfunction or low libido in men, as it improves blood circulation, while lowering blood pressure and anxiousness. It also contains chrysin, which actively helps raise/conserve testosterone levels. Other principles within passionflower tea may help elevate circulating testosterone by inhibition of aromatase activity within the body, thus preventing the conversion of testosterone to its metabolites.

Main medicinal actions: Analgesic, antidepressant, antispasmodic, anxiolytic, cardiotonic, diuretic, hypnotic, hypotensive, nervine, neuroprotective, opioidergic, sedative, testosterone booster, vasodilator.

Dosage

For insomnia, the recommendation is a strong cup one hour before bedtime. For anxiety and other therapeutics 2–3 cups during the day are advisable for treatment duration. For prolonged use, a weekend pause every two weeks is recommended.

Caution

Avoid in pregnancy and breastfeeding. May interact with anticonvulsants, anticoagulants, benzodiazepines, tricyclic antidepressants and prescription sedatives. Recurrent usage can aggravate conditions caused by excessive testosterone.

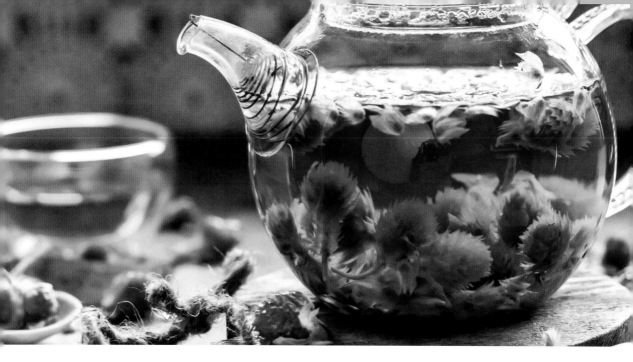

Red Clover Tea

(Trifolium pratense)

Botanical family
Leguminosae

Parts used
Aerial parts

Flavour profile
Sweet

Red clover is rich in phytoestrogens, calcium, iron, magnesium, manganese, niacin, phosphorus, potassium and selenium. Its beginnings in herbalism were as a popular spring tonic (a bitter) and as a purifying and drawing herb. Long utilised and then much studied and researched, it has been shown to support female health issues and be of benefit in certain cases of cancer.

How to make
While fresh herb is possible, in the main dried flowers and foliage are utilised to produce tea. The brew is best suited to a long infusion at 7–15 minutes, with a ratio of 1–2 tablespoons per cup of boiling water. It is traditionally made strong. Available in teabag and loose form. Some blends are comprised of dried flowers only, which yields a sweeter tea.

Health benefits
Historically utilised as a bitter tonic to excite some biliary secretion and augment the detoxification functions of the lymphatic system, lungs, liver and kidneys. Beneficial to treat acne, recurrent boils, eczema and

psoriasis. It is also used as a cooled topical wash for those conditions and to treat abscesses and ulcerations. The herb has a history in poultices and beverages to reduce mastitis and treat other breast inflammations.

Red clover is one of the richest sources of isoflavones – water-soluble phytoestrogens which mimic the activities of oestrogen when ingested. It has a long history of use to treat PMS and menopause-related symptoms – not just to reduce hot flushes, but also to control lipid profile and lessen arterial plaque that can arise post-menopause. Isoflavones and the plant's mineral content can also play a role in slowing osteoporosis, by helping to boost bone mineral density in pre- and peri-menopausal women. The tea is sometimes coined a natural HRT.

Phytoestrogens have potential in limiting the development of benign prostatic hyperplasia and are considered to be antimutagenic, antiproliferative and chemopreventive, but with the caveat that some cancers are oestrogen dependent and then the oestrogenic action would feed rather than weed. Clover also contains the phytoestrogens biochanin A and biochanin B (formononetin). Biochanin A is used in conventional medicine to address adenocarcinoma of the pancreas and pancreatic cancer, and is currently under evaluation as having a potential role in inhibiting the signalling pathways in HER-2-positive breast cancer cells. Biochanin B has been shown to have anticancer activity in colorectal cancer and prostate cancer, and to be a neuroprotective agent in Alzheimer's disease.

Main medicinal actions: Antimutagenic, antioxidant, antiproliferative, antiscrofulous, antispasmodic, aperient, chemopreventive, detox, expectorant, hypocholesterolaemic, oestrogenic, sedative.

Dosage
Therapeutic range is in the region of 1–3 cups daily for a set period, with a break and re-uptake cycle, until the issue resolves.

Caution
Avoid in pregnancy. Avoid with oestrogen-dependent tumours. Phytoestrogens can interfere with contraceptive medications. Avoid if on blood-thinning medication.

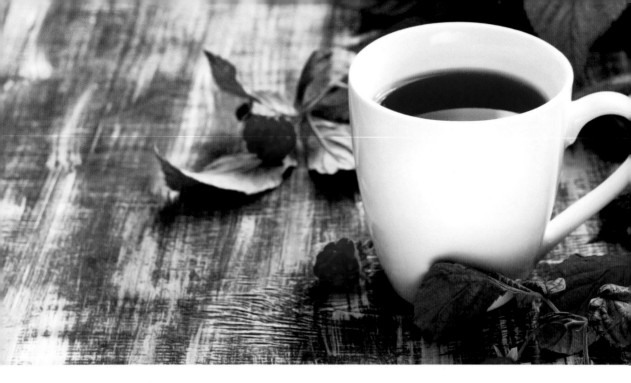

Red Raspberry Leaf Tea

(Rubus idaeus and *R. strigosus)*

Botanical family
Rosaceae

Parts used
Leaves

Flavour profile
Tannin

'Red' is in its common name here to distinguish from many other and lesser medicinal 'raspberries'. The herbal tea most researched and the one covered in this entry is sourced from cultivars or hybrids of *Rubus idaeus* and/or its red cousin *Rubus strigosus*.

How to make
The dried herbage is available in loose and teabag form. Suited to an infusion made with water fresh off the boil and a 5–7-minute steep time. A single teabag or a rounded teaspoon of herb per cup of water is the ideal ratio. Always use dried raspberry leaves as unprocessed fresh leaves can cause nausea. Pure leaf tea can taste bitter to tart and so is often sweetened to taste. Some proprietary blends on the market may mix with fruit pieces or other herbs such as hibiscus or rose to mellow the flavour.

Health benefits

Traditionally used around pregnancy and childbirth. The minerals and phytochemicals in the leaf help to strengthen the pelvic and uterine muscles in anticipation of pregnancy (prior to conception) and then are availed of again in the last trimester to trigger uterine relaxation and tonification in a manner supportive to a shorter labour. By improving the efficiency of pelvic and uterine muscles it has history as a remedy against pre-eclampsia, pre-term labour, prolonged labour, delayed labour and post-partum haemorrhage, as well as a role in post-partum recovery.

It also has a long-standing application in regulating the menstrual cycle and decreasing menstrual cramps. Being iron-rich, it has also been used to address anaemia. The foliage contains significant amounts of polyphenol antioxidants, which promote the health of cardiovascular and endothelial (blood and lymphatic) vessels. Raspberry leaf tea is also somewhat insulinogenic due to its chromium, magnesium and zinc content, and can help stabilise high blood-sugar levels.

As a cooled rinse, its astringent, antiseptic and anti-inflammatory principles make it very effective in treating oral infections, including gingivitis, cankers and cuts. It also has a tradition as an eyewash for sties and conjunctivitis, and in gargling for tonsillitis and sore throats.

Main medicinal actions: Analgesic, antibacterial, antidiarrhoeal, antiemetic, anti-inflammatory, antiseptic, astringent, birthing aid, cholagogue, decongestant, diaphoretic, diuretic, hypoglycaemic, oestrogenic, ophthalmic, uterine tonic.

Dosage

1 cup daily is generally recommended. Upper limit is 2 cups.

Caution

In relation to pregnancy, it is generally recommended for use prior to conception and during the last three months of pregnancy. The phytochemical make-up of raspberry leaf in higher or prolonged doses can alter oestrogen metabolism, which on an individual basis may lessen or worsen oestrogen-related illnesses. Supervision required.

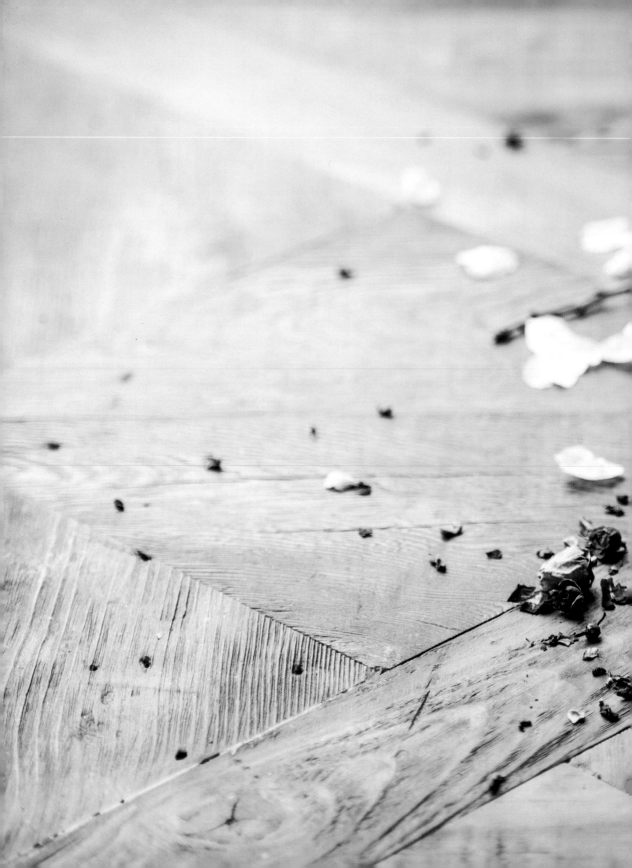

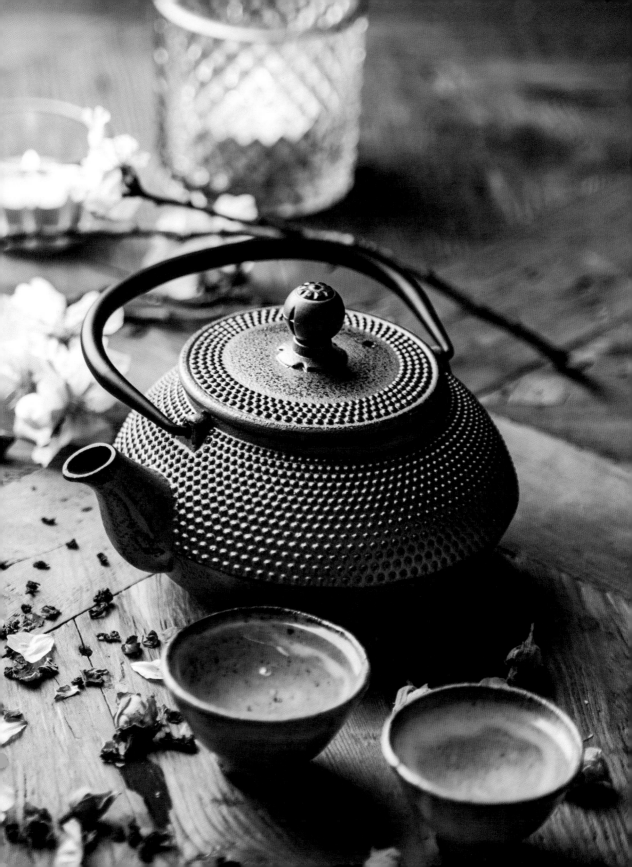

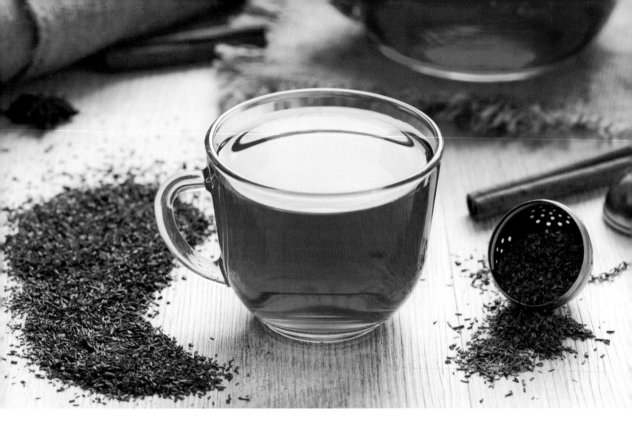

Rooibos Tea

(Aspalathus linearis)

Botanical family
Fabaceae

Parts used
Leaves and twigs

Flavour profile
Sweet

Rooibos means 'red bush'. Traditionally it was a medicinal herb in South Africa. Its global popularity came about first via rebranding it as a refreshing alternative to black tea when, in 1904, a local harvester, Benjamin Ginsberg, began to market it as 'mountain tea'. Later, it became known as Red Bush or South African red tea. Rooibos is processed in a manner similar to black tea: its leaves and twigs are harvested, bruised to instigate enzymatic oxidation and then dried. Compared to black tea, however, it has lower tannin levels and no caffeine.

How to make
Best via an infusion of boiling water in a lidded teapot, or by placing the saucer over the cup for a 3–7 minute duration. The standard ratio is 1 teaspoon of dried, finely chopped herb or 1 teabag per cup. Rooibos is one of those rare herbal teas that may be taken with milk. It is pleasant straight up (sweet and even fruity) and many regular drinkers who opt

for extra sweetness favour the traditional lemon and honey. A longer brew can alter flavour to astringent notes. Can be served cooled or even iced.

Health benefits

Popular as a carminative and anti-colic beverage, due in part to its many flavonoid glycosides and their anti-inflammatory and antispasmodic principles. It is soothing to nausea, heartburn, intestinal upset and also to muscle cramping. Being antibacterial and antiviral, it has form in treating upset stomachs, including those caused by rotaviruses. The tea's antiviral activity extends to colds, flu and other viral conditions.

Packed full of antioxidants – close to forty different varieties – two in particular are of interest: aspalathin and nothofagin. Aspalathin is exclusive to the redbush plant and apart from preventing oxidative stress and actively scavenging free radicals, it improves the metabolism of glucose and helps boost insulin secretion from the pancreas, making it of benefit for diabetics. But by improving insulin resistance it may also have a role in other conditions affected by poor glucose absorption, from tinnitus to polycystic ovary syndrome. Nothofagin inhibits glucose-induced vascular inflammation and can help impede the initiation and progression of atherosclerosis, as well as slow diabetic neuropathy and other diabetic complications.

Rutin present in the tea helps prevent the formation of blood clots, and its content of chrysoeriol and orientin improves vascular health and supports circulation.

Main medicinal actions: Anti-allergenic, anti-inflammatory, antioxidant, antispasmodic, bronchial dilator, carminative, digestive, hypoglycaemic, hypotensive, oestrogenic, skin tonic, vasoprotective.

Dosage

Upper limits of 2–4 cups daily.

Caution

Avoid in early pregnancy. Caution if dealing with oestrogen dominance or hormone-sensitive health conditions. Rooibos tea can impede the absorption of iron so best limited or avoided if anaemic.

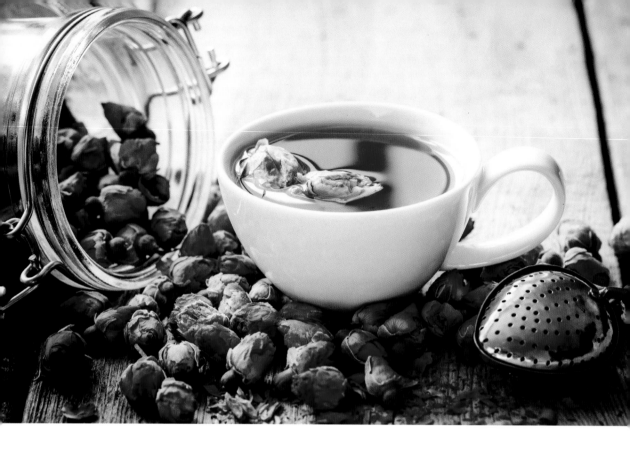

Rose Petal/Rosebud Tea

(*Rosa rugosa* and select species)

Botanical family
Rosaceae

Parts used
Petals/flower buds

Flavour profile
Floral, fruity

Rosa rugosa is most commonly utilised as a source of rose tea but other species include *Rosa canina*, *Rosa damascena*, *Rosa laevigata* and *Rosa gallica* var. *centifolia*. As rose petals and rose buds have the same healing action, the details here are interchangeable.

How to make
To maximise the vitamin C and other antioxidant agents it is best to rest boiled water for 30–60 seconds before making an infusion. Fresh petals will need the bitter white portion at the base of the petal removed; dried petals are good to go. The standard ratio is 1–2 teaspoons per cup required. As roses contain many favourable and bioactive volatile oils, it is good to make in a teapot or covered cup. Infusion duration is 3–5 minutes. Can be sweetened with some honey or stevia. Suitable for cooling and serving over ice.

Health benefits

Rose tea has a history of use as a cooling beverage to remedy menopausal hot flushes and night sweats, and, in its sedative and nervine actions, to address irritability, mental and physical fatigue, and also mild depression. Its oldest tradition is to relieve uterine and menstrual irregularities and to attenuate PMS. Certainly its supply of calcium, iron, manganese, magnesium and B vitamins are of benefit, as are the flavonoids that contribute to improved blood flow.

Rose petals store a good quantity of vitamin C, making this tea immune boosting and system cleansing. It has a good reputation in supporting viral illness recovery and for general pick-me-up applications. It also contains significant amounts of polyphenols that actively repair cellular damage and act as free-radical scavengers, contributing to its association as a rejuvenating tonic. Polyphenols also exert an influence on gut bacteria and on the chemistry of inflammation, and further help reduce the effect of bacterial and viral infection.

Rose stimulates bile and is viewed as a detox and digestive. Its antimicrobial nature is beneficial to gut health and to urinary tract health. Rose tea shows some antimicrobial activity against *Staphylococcus epidermidis, S. aureus, Escherichia coli, Bacillus subtilis, Micrococcus luteus, Klebsiella pneumoniae, Pseudomonas aeruginosa, Proteus mirabilis* and also against two significant yeast strains: *Candida albicans* and *C. parapsilosis.*

Main medicinal actions: Antibacterial, antidepressant, anti-inflammatory, antiseptic, antispasmodic, antiviral, aphrodisiac, astringent, blood tonic, detox, digestive, diuretic, emmenagogue, expectorant, febrifuge, nervine, sedative, uterine.

Dosage

The standard range is 1–2 cups daily over therapeutic duration. Over-consumption can cause nausea or headache.

Caution

Avoid in pregnancy due to uterine activity. Avoid recurrent use if on blood-thinning medication.

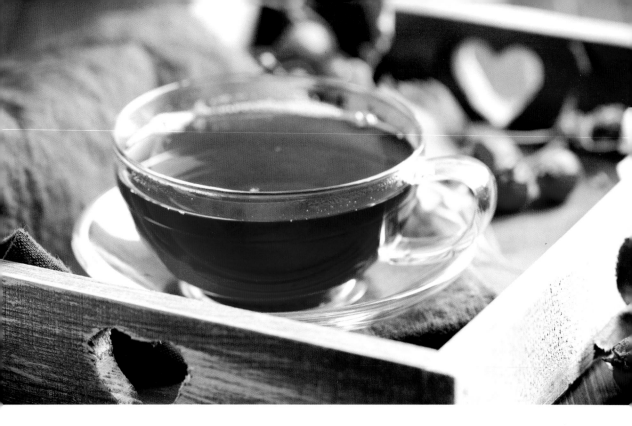

Rosehip Tea

*(Rosa canina, R. laevigata, R. rugosa
and R. rubiginosa)*

Botanical family
Rosaceae

Parts used
Fruit (hip)

Flavour profile
Tangy

Roses and apples share the same botanical family and their fruits have been keeping doctors away for as long as idioms have existed. Rosehips feature in the earliest herbal and the oldest medicinal texts, in the main as a general health tonic and as convalescence support, but also to ease a whole variety of illness symptoms.

How to make
If using rosehips from a forage, do note that the inner seeds contain bitter and irritant hairs that require removal before use. The easiest way is to slice the hips lengthways and simply scoop them out with a knife. Hips can be utilised fresh or dried for later use. Hip tea can be served hot or iced. It is tart and will need sweetening. Old recipes call for a lot of sugar, but a pinch of stevia will do the trick.

Teabags can be infused for 3–5 minutes in boiling or post-boil water.

Fresh and dried hips need some coaxing to release their flavour and phytochemicals, and so are traditionally decocted. Old recipes would have recommended half an hour or more – but you can add to cold water and bring to a slow boil, then simmer for 5 minutes before resting for a further 5–10 minutes. The ratio is 1–2 teaspoons of chopped hip per cup. The dried hips often have a stronger taste.

Health benefits

Traditionally employed to treat colds, flu, coughs, mucous congestion, fevers and both bacterial and viral infections. The tea promotes light perspiration and urine flow, and so helps eliminate toxins and cleanses the body, boosting our own inherent healing potential and recovery time. The tea has a reputation for cooling menopausal hot flushes and reducing profuse night sweats. Its content of isoflavone phytoestrogens can act as a mild HRT.

The ability of bioflavonoids within the fruit to promote good general health is not to be underestimated, and they also perform a role in supporting cardiovascular health and addressing circulatory difficulties from varicose veins to erectile dysfunction. The presence of vitamin P in rosehips further enhances the functioning of the capillaries and peripheral blood circulation. Rosehip tea can also slightly thin blood to improve flow. Externally the cooled tea is popular as a skin cleanser and toner, and its antimicrobial action is great for acne and breakouts.

Main medicinal actions: Analgesic, anti-inflammatory, antimicrobial, astringent, carminative, circulatory tonic, decongestant, diaphoretic, digestive, emmenagogue, febrifuge, laxative, nervine, stimulant, vasotonic.

Dosage

The general protocol is a daily cup for general well-being and 2–3 cups as therapeutic to ailments.

Caution

Generally regarded as safe, but note that it can have oestrogenic, blood-thinning and iron accumulation effects, which may be relevant to some clinical illnesses and medications.

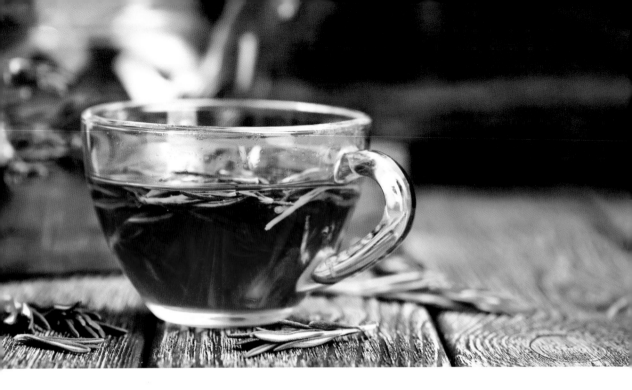

Rosemary Tea

(Rosmarinus officinalis)

Botanical family
Lamiaceae

Parts used
Leaves and stems

Flavour profile
Balsamic/pine-like

The Latin genus name *Rosmarinus* is derived from *ros*, denoting 'dew', and *marinus* – 'of the sea'. Many assume that the shade of blue of the flower inspired this. There may also be a 'sacred plant' link to Aphrodite, who emerged from the sea – her devotees were said to utilise the plant as a sexual health tonic.

How to make
The volatile oils contain a lot of healing so it is best to make rosemary tea with water that has moved off boiling temperature and in a teapot or covered cup to trap those molecules in the drinking liquid and not allow them to evaporate in the steam. Standard ratio is 1–2 teaspoons per cup and a 3–7-minute infusion.

Health benefits
Rosemary is a digestive support, stimulating appetite and the secretion of gastric juices, and helps to address dyspeptic and gastric complaints. It is effective in encouraging the efficient digestion of fats and improves

the elimination of toxins. Its antibacterial and antifungal properties keep the digestive system cleansed and healthy.

Several of its volatile oils stimulate blood flow to the brain and support acetylcholine levels that function within our system. Acetylcholine is a neurotransmitter servicing both excitatory and inhibitory functions, i.e. it can slow or speed up nerve signals to better serve our health needs. Acetylcholine also increases the modification of synapses and acts upon the hippocampus – so apart from improved cognitive function, its synaptic interventions make it a tool against depression, dementia and Alzheimer's.

Rosemary's potently antioxidant diterpenes and the presence of apigenin deliver anxiolytic and antidepressant-like effects. Rosemary is also a brilliant circulatory stimulant and venotonic, which can be utilised to address hypotension and venous insufficiency. It contains good quantities of hesperidin and diosmin, which help capillary fragility and improve peripheral blood flow.

Rosmarinic acid is a powerful analgesic and anti-inflammatory compound and, with rosemary's ursolic acid and apigenin content, validate rosemary as a pain suppressant to cramps, muscle spasms, rheumatism and also intercostal neuralgia. Cooled rosemary tea is also antimicrobial and has a role to treat acne and skin outbreaks, as well as dandruff.

Main medicinal actions: Adrenal support, antidepressant, anti-inflammatory, antioxidant, antiseptic, antispasmodic, astringent, capillary tonic, cardiotonic, carminative, cholagogue, circulatory stimulant, decongestant, diaphoretic, diuretic, emmenagogue, hepatoprotective, nervine, nervous system relaxant, restorative, sedative, uterine stimulant, venotonic.

Dosage
Generally in the range of 1–2 cups daily for treatment duration, upper limit of 3 cups. Overuse can cause nausea.

Caution
Avoid in pregnancy or if utilising anticoagulation or antiplatelet medication.

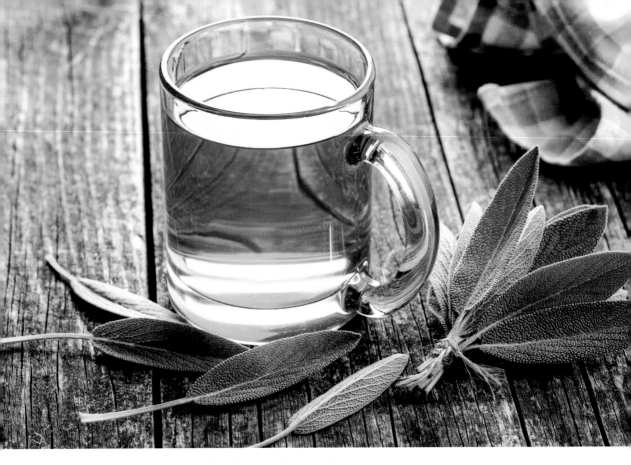

Sage Tea

(Salvia officinalis)

Botanical family
Lamiaceae

Parts used
Leaves

Flavour profile
Earthy, sweet, with peppery or bitter notes

Both the names sage and *salvia* are etymologically linked to 'save', denoting its manifold medicinal applications. *Officinalis* further reminds us of its official curative status – from a time in herbal history when there were official herbs and non-validated herbs.

How to make
The tradition is to put 1 teabag, or 1 teaspoon of fresh chopped, or 1–2 teaspoons of dried and crumbled sage leaves per cup into a lidded tea pot and add boiled water that has rested from the boiling point for 30–60 seconds. The rested temperature does not destroy any of the volatile oils and the teapot restrains them from evaporation. You can also cover a cup with a saucer to hold onto the volatile oils. General infusion time is 5–7 minutes. Sweeten to taste.

Health benefits

Sage has many health applications, from bronchial support to gastro-protective, but it is perhaps best known as a female tonic – having oestrogenic and emmenagogue actions beneficial to menstrual and menopause complaints. Its anti-inflammatory and antispasmodic constituents, such as rosmarinic acid, help relieve stomach cramps and mild back pain. Rosmarinic acid also helps reduce anxiety and nervous tension, while sage's content of linalool has sedative properties.

Sage tea contains phytosterols that exert a cooling action upon the body and, being an antihydrotic/depurative herb, it further helps to re-duce or prevent sweating and offers some benefit to alleviating the night sweats associated with menopause. This action is also availed of to stop lactation post-weaning. Phytosterols also inhibit cholesterol absorption.

Sage tea actually helps lower blood glucose levels in a manner similar to the diabetic drug Metformin. The sundry flavonoids and phe-nolic acids of sage also show potential in treatment of hyperlipidaemia – a metabolic disorder contributing to co-occurring conditions of dia-betes, atherosclerosis, cardiovascular and cerebrovascular diseases. One agent – carnosic acid – is known to increase blood circulation, particularly in the brain, where it also acts to help prevent neuro-degenerative damage.

Externally, cooled sage tea can be used as an antibacterial mouth-wash and as a gargle for sore throats and tonsillitis.

Main medicinal actions: Analgesic, antihydrotic, antihyperlipidaemic, anti-inflammatory, antimicrobial, antioxidant, antiseptic, antispasmodic, astringent, bitter tonic, carminative, cholagogue, depurative, diabetic support, digestive, diuretic, emmenagogue, oestrogenic, vasodilator.

Dosage

Generally kept within the limit of 1 or 2 cups per day.

Caution

Be aware of its oestrogenic actions. Avoid in pregnancy and breastfeeding. Avoid with epilepsy as its thujone content can trigger epileptic attacks. Can increase the effects of sedative, diabetic and blood-pressure medication.

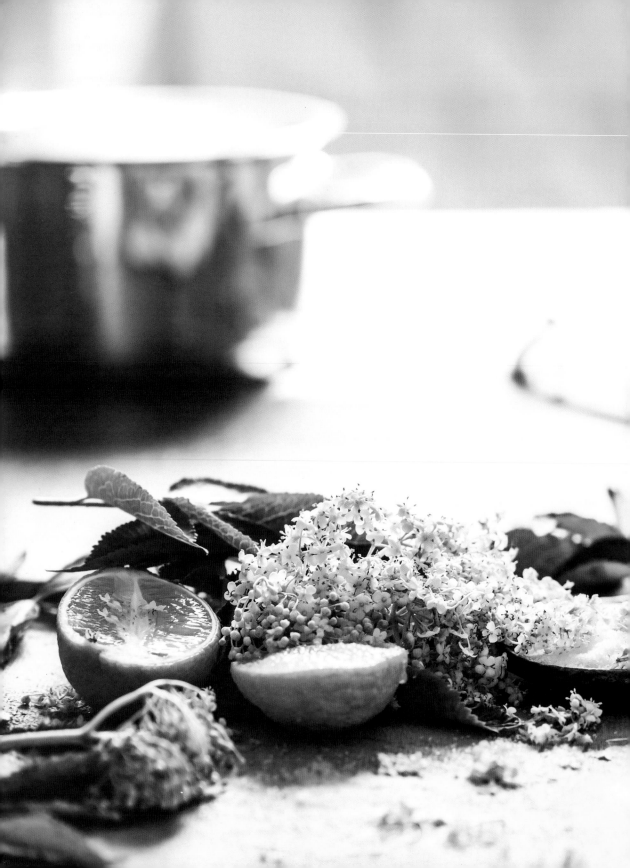

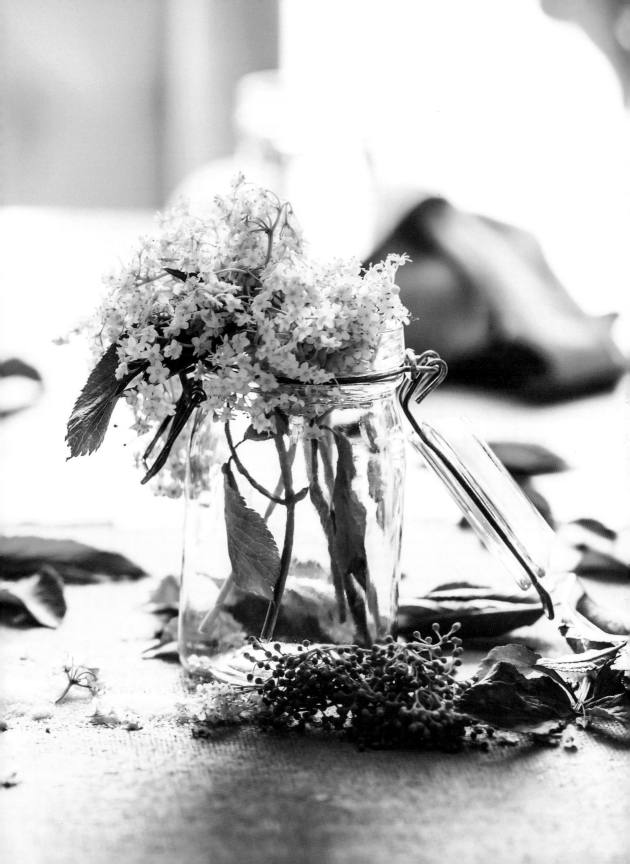

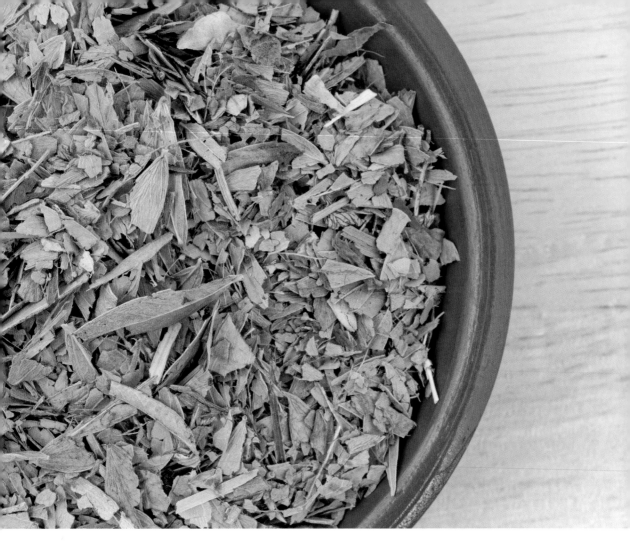

Senna Tea

(Cassia senna and
C. angustifolia syn. *Senna alexandrina)*

Botanical family
Leguminosae

Parts used
Leaves and pods

Flavour profile
Bitter

Senna is a strictly medicinal tea with a very definite purpose – to be a cathartic (a strong laxative). Senna extracts feature in modern medications, including as a preparation taken prior to undergoing a colonoscopy. It does feature in some of the more potent 'detox teas', but is also readily available as a loose herb and herbal teabag, and so rightly features here. However, to be clear, I would not advise it to be used as a detox or weight loss aid.

How to make

Once the popularity was for a traditional cold infusion with 4–8 dried pods steeped in cold water overnight (6–12 hours). Contemporary blends and teabag versions include leaf and pod and are suited to a standard infusion of boiling water and a steepage time of 10–15 minutes, before straining and consuming.

If in loose form, ½ to 1 teaspoon is general. The taste is bitter, but it is often brewed/mixed with carminative herbs such as fennel, chamomile, etc., to lessen griping and sweeten the tea. Can also be sweetened with honey.

Health benefits

It's considered a bit of a one-trick pony, but it achieves that trick to a high standard: the ultimate remedy to chronic constipation, whereby the anthraquinones in the senna leaf and pods stimulate contraction of the large intestine and colon muscle and so instigate a bowel movement.

Turns out it has a second trick, however. Senna tea also has applications topically – to inhibit the growth and proliferation of bacteria, fungi and parasites. It features in some old herbals as a remedy to acne, athlete's foot and ringworm.

Main medicinal actions: Antibacterial, cathartic, colon-cleansing.

Dosage

Senna is not for long-term use and is best limited to short period usage – no more than 7 days. Senna is strong acting and is best begun at the lowest dose possible so as to allay any unpleasant effects – so try a few sips, at first, then graduate to half a cup, then a full cup if required. It can at times be slow acting, so be patient and expect a 6–12-hour delay before it starts working.

Caution

Excessive consumption or recurrent use may cause electrolyte imbalances, abdominal cramps, nausea and vomiting. Not advised with digestive illnesses such as Crohn's, IBS, etc. Not advised in pregnancy or nursing. Also, due to its effects and a resultant dramatic decrease in transit time, it can interfere with absorption of prescription medication.

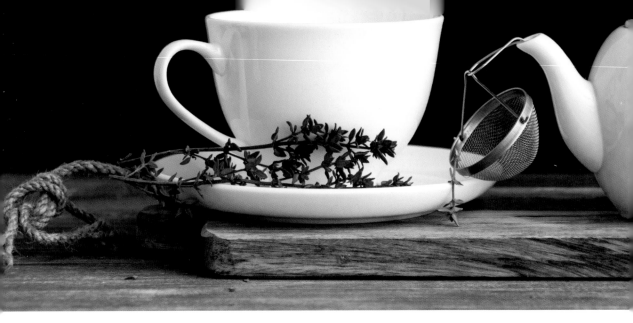

Thyme Tea

(*Thymus vulgaris*)

Botanical family
Laminaceae

Parts used
Aerial parts

Flavour profile
Earthy

Common thyme (*Thymus vulgaris*) is the most common form of thyme tea. It can be sourced in teabag form, made from the dried herb on your spice rack, or availed of from garden-grown plants. Other garden varieties include lemon thyme (*Thymus x citriodorus*), orange-scented thyme (*Thymus 'fragrantissimus'*), coconut thyme (*Thymus Coccineus*) and caraway thyme (*Thymus herba-barona*).

How to make
A thyme infusion can be produced from fresh or dried herbage – generally at a ratio per cup of 1–2 teaspoons fresh, though less if dry. As with all volatile oil tea, brew with boiled water rested for 30–60 seconds in a covered cup or lidded pot. Standard infusion times are 3–7 minutes. Longer length brews can take on a more bitter taste. The flavour profile of thyme is in the earthy range but, depending upon the variety, it can be more piney or peppery and with an accent of citrus or mint-like notes.

Health benefits

Thyme is full of neuroactive and antioxidant flavonoids, prompting its usage to slow the progression of cancer, dementia, cardiovascular disease and even ageing. Many of these flavonoids also interact with the brain's GABA receptors and can influence mood and cognitive functioning. Apigenin, for example, increases brain connections and lifts mood; luteolin decreases 'brain fog' and regulates brain expression of pro-inflammatory genes/molecules.

Thyme's volatile oils – notably thymol and carvacrol – are highly effective biocides that seek and destroy harmful organisms of fungal, bacterial and viral infections, but which also help activate a more efficient immune response to those infections. Thyme promotes white blood cell formation whilst raising the effectiveness of macrophages (a type of white blood cell that engulfs and digests foreign bodies and cellular debris) in tracking and killing invading organisms. Utilised to treat candida, digestive upset and food poisoning, and in fighting colds and flu and other infections.

Thyme has a long history in treating asthma, whooping cough, bronchitis, sinus, hay fever, pneumonia and pleurisy, helping to strengthen and dilate the respiratory tract and expectorate phlegm. Externally a cooled thyme tea is a wound healer and skin tonic for acne, eczema and psoriasis. It also makes a great gargle for mouth and throat infections and pains.

Main medicinal actions: Analgesic, antibacterial, anticancer, antifungal, antihelmintic, antioxidant, antiseptic, antispasmodic, antitussive, anti-viral, astringent, carminative, decongestant, diaphoretic, disinfectant, expectorant, mood enhancing, nervine, secretolitic, uterine stimulant, vasodilator.

Dosage

A daily cup is prophylactic. Therapeutically, it is advisable to observe the upper limit of 3–4 cups daily for the duration of the treatment.

Caution

Thyme is a potent herb and overuse can cause some gastric upset. Avoid in pregnancy due to potential uterine stimulation.

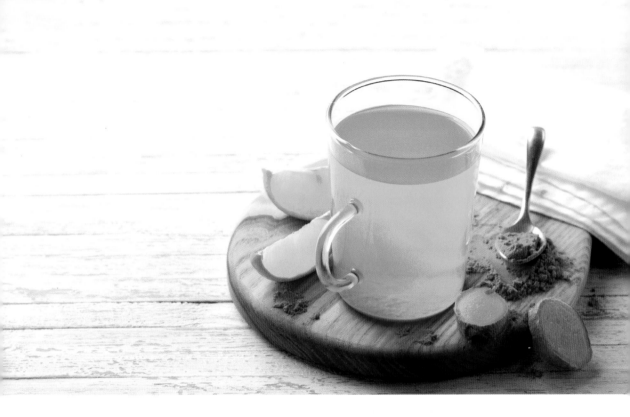

Turmeric Tea

(Curcuma longa)

Botanical family
Zingiberaceae

Parts used
Roots/powdered spice

Flavour profile
Bitter spice

Turmeric is one of the most widely researched spices in the world and validated as a healing agent of strong repute. Some brands of turmeric tea are actually a green tea flavoured with turmeric or a mix of turmeric spice with various roots and herbs. The healing attributes and cautions of those teas would be different to pure turmeric tea. This entry relates to a single, pure ingredient tea.

How to make
½–1 teaspoon of ground spice can be infused in boiling water for 5 minutes. Older traditions decocted the sliced chopped root for 10–15 minutes – generally 1 teaspoon per cup. There is also a tradition of decocting it in milk to enhance the solubility/bioavailability of the curcumin content, which is more readily fat-soluble. A warm milk infusion of the ground spice is also possible.

Health benefits

Turmeric has myriad healing applications, from skin tonic to liver and digestive complaints. It features prominently in folk medicine as a means of addressing female health issues, and has wide appeal as a tonic for convalescence and as a prophylactic for viral and bacterial infections. A lot of its attributes come from curcumin – the polyphenolic compound that pigments the root.

Curcumin amps up the process of conversion of cholesterol into bile acids and it exerts anti-inflammatory and antioxidant effects on a par with, if not superior to, those of hydrocortisone. Curcumin actively inhibits the formation of beta-amyloid and other plaque-like agents that obstruct normal cerebral function in dementia. Turmeric's chemicals help bolster levels of the brain-derived neurotrophic factor – a brain hormone which supports the growth of new neurons and combats various degenerative processes in the brain.

Curcumin also actively inhibits an enzyme known as topoisomerase, which is required for the replication of cancer cells, and it further inhibits the expression of the nuclear factor B (NFB) responsible for invasion, tumour angiogenesis and metastasis. Turmeric may also help alter a cancer cell's resistance to chemotherapy and its mechanism of shielding from our innate immune system's 'search and destroy' mechanisms.

Main medicinal actions: Anti-arthritic, antibiotic, anticancer, anti-inflammatory, anti-ischaemic, antimicrobial, antioxidant, carminative, cholagogue, circulatory stimulant, digestive, oestrogenic, hepato-protective, hypolipidaemic, uterine stimulant.

Dosage

In general health 1 cup per day is supportive. Therapeutically, the advisement is in the range of 2–3 cups daily for treatment duration or 400–600mg of pure turmeric powder/spice 3 times daily.

Caution

Avoid in pregnancy and with oestrogen-implicated illnesses such as endometriosis/uterine fibroids, ovarian and breast cancers. Contra-indicated with hyperacidity, GERD, stomach ulcers, biliary obstruction and gallstones. May impact upon blood-thinning medication.

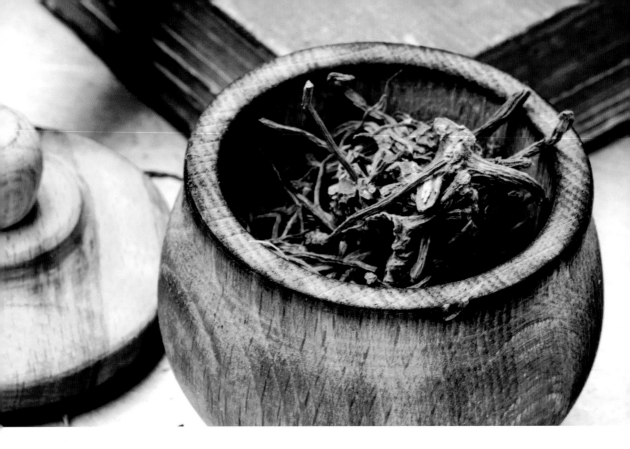

Valerian Tea

(*Valeriana officinalis*)

Botanical family
Valerianaceae

Parts used
Roots

Flavour profile
Acrid

While *officinalis* denotes an 'officially sanctioned herb', valerian may derive from the Latin word *valere*, meaning to prevail or to be strong/healthy. It has a long history in herbalism.

How to make

A standard infusion of a single teabag or 2 teaspoons of chopped dried root per cup. Often pot made – to contain the strong musky aroma – with boiling water and a 5-minute steepage. Optionally, some herbalists prefer a cold infusion of similar ratios, which would then be allowed to stand for 6–8 hours.

To put it politely the aroma and taste is strong and may lean towards sweaty rather than musky to some nasal receptors and taste buds. Some stevia or honey may sweeten the deal. Often consumed cold as that way it is easier to quickly swallow.

Health benefits

Valerian is often spoken of as a 'natural valium'. It is most utilised as a night-time sleep aid and daytime relaxant. The valerenic acid and valepotriates that it contains exhibit sedative actions via several routes, but their impact upon GABA is interesting.

GABA is an inhibitory neurotransmitter, which slows down signals between neurons, prompting more relaxed states, physiologically and mentally. The constituents of valerian not only bind to GABA receptors, thereby simulating a surge in 'slow down' signals, but also prompt the production and release of GABA, as well as inhibiting degradation of existing GABA. Valerian itself contains small amounts of GABA. This three-fold push into sedation is what makes it a superior treatment for disturbed sleep patterns and a natural regulator of responses to stressful stimuli.

Valepotriates act on the same brain chemistry in the same way as the pharmacological medications used to treat generalised anxiety disorder. Some herbalists would also utilise valerian tea to attenuate the withdrawal symptoms from addictive substances. Valepotriates are also antispasmodic, and valerian tea therefore has a history in treating cramps, muscle spasm and various neuralgias. In recent years it has become popular to take the edge off fibromyalgia, Lyme disease and other chronic illnesses that are exacerbated by both poor night-time sleep and daytime stresses.

Main medicinal actions: Analgesic, antibiotic, antispasmodic, anxiolytic, bitter, carminative, emmenagogue, expectorant, hypnotic, hypotensive, nervous system relaxant, sedative.

Dosage

Traditionally a cup 30–60 minutes before bedtime for insomnia, anxiety and other uses. The upper limit is 2–3 times daily.

Caution

Not recommended in pregnancy or nursing. Recurrent use of valerian can potentially increase the effect of prescription medicines targeting anxiety, insomnia, depression and convulsions.

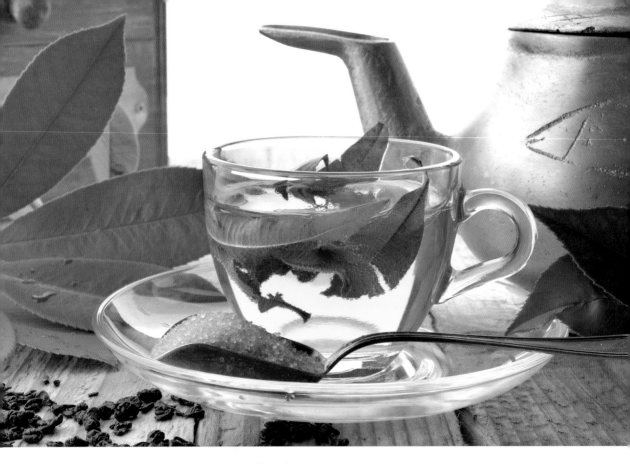

Vervain Tea

(*Verbena officinalis*)

Botanical family
Verbenaceae

Parts used
Aerial parts

Flavour profile
Strong, bitter

The name 'verbena' has historically been utilised to denote 'altar plants', but vervain also has a very physical role as a medicinal plant to remedy gallstones and kidney and bladder irritations. The etymology of the word likely derives from the Celtic *ferfaen*, combining *fer* (to drive away) and *faen* (a stone).

How to make

This is an interesting one, as how you prepare it alters its application. For example, simmering decoctions at boiling point for 1–2 minutes will diminish/destroy the stimulant principles and turn it into a more nervine and sedate beverage. Infusion via hot water previously boiled but rested for a minute, however, will extract the more stimulant nature. The best ratio for both is 1 teaspoon of dried or 2 teaspoons of fresh per cup. It is bitter by any delivery method, but can be improved with sweetening.

Health benefits

The bitter quality makes for a strong digestive tonic that not only increases bile secretion and pancreatic enzymes, but actively triggers salivation and improves intestinal motility. It has a long history in treating poor appetite during chronic illness or slow convalescence, and also in improving liver function, treating gallstones, urinary gravel and infections of the bladder.

Vervain is lauded as a sleep aid – its polyphenol verbascoside helps shorten how long it takes to fall asleep while also helping to increase the duration of sleep. Traditionally, it has been used as a nerve restorative and recuperative herb, and to alleviate psychological states of anxiety, irritability and nervous tension. It has history as a female tonic to reduce menstrual cramping and, in its stimulant form, as an emmenagogue to tone the uterus after childbirth or in advance of conception.

Vervain contains two interesting antioxidants: caffeic acid, which is beneficial in the relieving of muscular pain and exercise-related fatigue, and lupeol, which has anti-inflammatory, antihyperglycaemic, and antimutagenic effects. The tea also supplies ursolic acid, which, among other positive health benefits, actively enhances Insulin-Like Growth Factor 1, which has a role in lessening lipids and blood glucose levels, but which also works with growth hormones to reproduce and regenerate cells.

Main medicinal actions: Analgesic, antidepressant, anti-inflammatory, antispasmodic, astringent, bitter, cholagogue, digestive, diaphoretic, diuretic, emmenagogue, galactagogue, hepatic stimulant, hypo-glycaemic, nervine, nervous system tonic, soothing, stimulant, uterine stimulant.

Dosage

Therapeutic dosages are generally in the range of 2–3 cups a day.

Caution

Avoid in the first two trimesters of pregnancy.

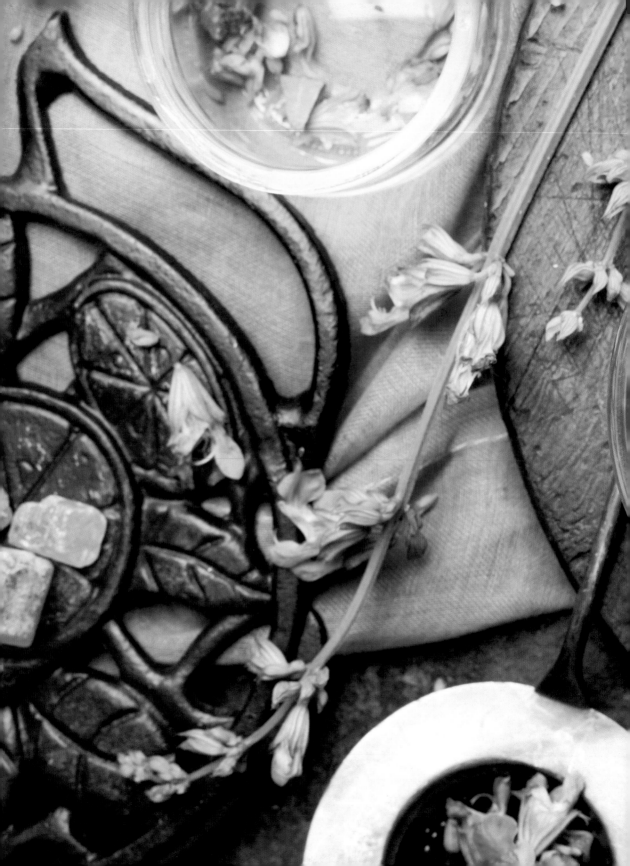

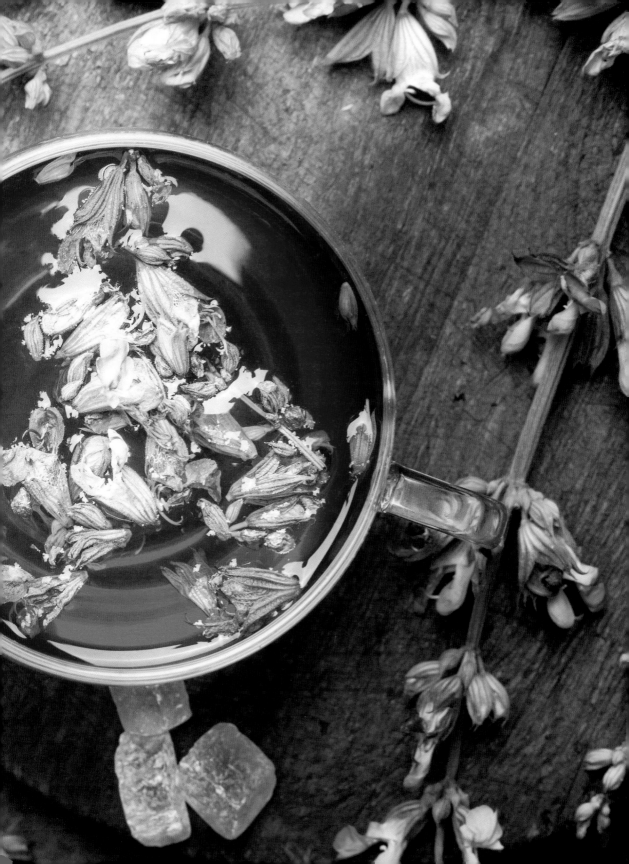

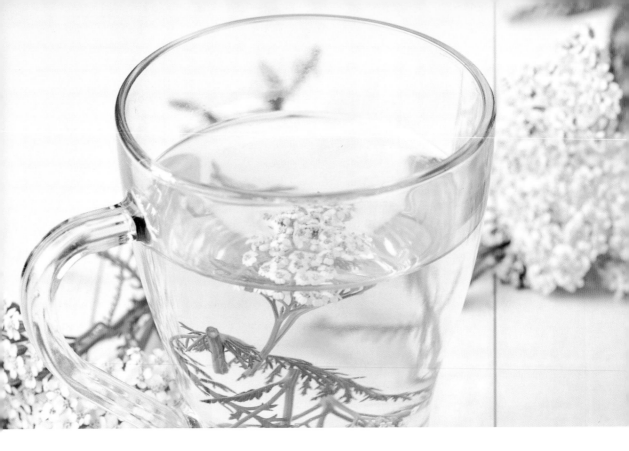

Yarrow Tea

(Achillea millefolium)

Botanical family
Asteraceae

Parts used
Aerial parts

Flavour profile
Sweetish, with tannin notes

Named for the Greek hero Achilles, who legend has it was either bathed in yarrow everyday by his mother to make him invincible, or discovered the medicinal uses of the plant and administered it to heal the wounds of his soldiers between charges and assaults at the Battle of Troy.

How to make
A single teabag or 1–2 teaspoons of fresh or dried herb per cup. In general, it is availed of via a standard infusion of 3–7 minutes after the addition of boiling water, but I would argue that to maintain the volatile oils content, you should rest the boiled water for 30 seconds and cover the cup with a saucer to trap the molecules inside the cup. Its astringency can increase with the longer duration of steepage. It is a pleasant-tasting tea, but for some palates its astringency – especially with the fresh herb – can call for some added sweetening.

Health benefits

Topically utilised as a styptic and skin tonic, the salicylic acid content within yarrow is analgesic and its tannins make it strongly astringent. Other constituents are antimicrobial and speed healing. Internally, yarrow is most often utilised as a bitter tonic that helps stimulate more efficient digestion, as its carminative, anti-inflammatory and antispasmodic effects make it suitable for the gamut of stomach upsets. It also eases menstrual cramps and attenuates symptoms of PMS and menopause.

The apigenin found in yarrow is potently anti-inflammatory and antispasmodic, and has a mild antidepressant and anti-stress impact. Its portion of azulene (also present in chamomile) delivers mind-calming as well as antispasmodic benefits. Yarrow has long been utilised to improve pelvic circulation and to stimulate the uterus and encourage menstruation. As a diaphoretic, it is helpful to reduce fevers and also to detox the body. Its capacity to help expel toxins has seen a tradition of use whereby it is said to clear eruptive infections such as measles and chickenpox.

Main medicinal actions: Analgesic, antihistamine, anti-inflammatory, antimicrobial, antispasmodic, astringent, bitter tonic, carminative, decongestant, diaphoretic, digestive, diuretic, emmenagogue, expectorant, haemostatic, hepatoprotective, hypotensive, nervine, uterine tonic, vasodilator, vasoprotective, vulnerary.

Dosage

Traditionally in the range of 2–3 cups per day for therapeutic purposes. If intended for long-term use over a few months, then single cups may be the preferred choice.

Caution

Avoid in pregnancy and if allergic to ragweed. Recurrent use can increase risk of photosensitivity. Long-term use without breaks is not advised as yarrow contains coumarins, which are known for their blood-thinning abilities, as well as small amounts of thujone, which can be toxic in large amounts or narcotic after prolonged use.

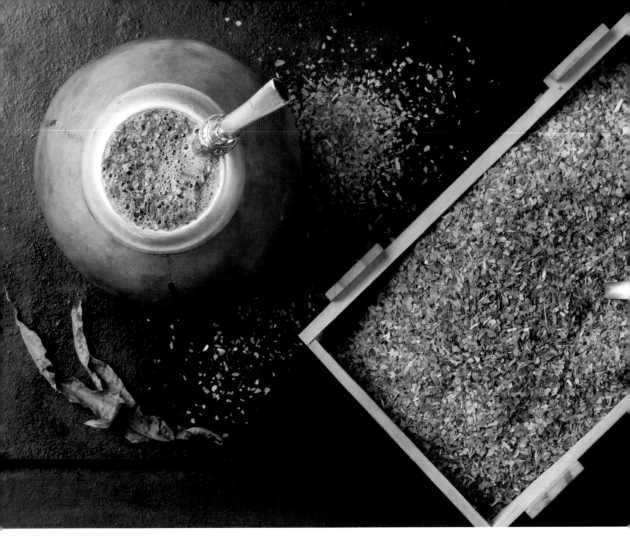

Yerba Mate Tea

(Ilex paraguariensis)

Botanical family
Aquifoliaceae

Parts used
Leaves

Flavour profile
Tannin to bitter

A pleasant and popular stimulant tea (the leaf contains caffeine) from South America and Paraguay in particular – as 'paraguar-iensis' denotes. Yerba has an etymological connection to the Spanish (*hierba*) and Portuguese (*erva*) words for herb, while the mate part derives from the indigenous Quechua languages and translates roughly as 'infusion herb'.

How to make
The best method is to pre-boil the water and let it cool for 1 minute

before using it to infuse the herb – the hotter the water the more bitter the taste, the longer the steepage the stronger the taste. The pre-boil removes some chemicals from tap water that can alter the uptake or taste of phytoconstituents. Available in teabag and also loose form, for which use 1 teaspoon per cup. Infusion length is recommended at 4–8 minutes. Can be chilled as an iced tea or reheated.

Health benefits

Commonly utilised as an uplifting and recuperative tea – it boosts energy levels and mental alertness, but also supports the aerobic breakdown of carbohydrates during exertion and helps delay the build-up of lactic acid. It encourages the production of corticosteroids, which provide relief to strained and inflamed areas of the body. Yerba mate is beneficial to both gym workouts and to allergy support, in that it helps to open respiratory pathways and bolster breathing capacity.

As for yerba mate's reputation in weight loss – its stimulant nature may suppress hunger, as its efficiency boost to carbohydrate metabolism means you draw more energy from the food you do eat and, feeling fuller, you are less likely to snack between meals. The broad array of flavonoids and phenolic acids within yerba mate also inhibit enzymes (including pancreatic lipase) which play a role in fat and cholesterol metabolism, and can help decrease fat storage.

Main medicinal actions: Anti-allergenic, antibacterial, anti-inflammatory, antioxidant, digestive, diuretic, febrifuge, hypocholesterolaemic, immune support, stimulant, weight management.

Dosage

Because it is caffeinated, it is recommended to not exceed 3 cups per day.

Caution

Can increase bile and stomach acids, which normally would support more efficient digestion but may, in some cases, exacerbate conditions such as GERD and other reflux disorders. Overuse can result in symptoms associated with caffeine overload: from restlessness to insomnia and increased heart rate to tremors.

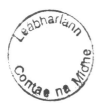

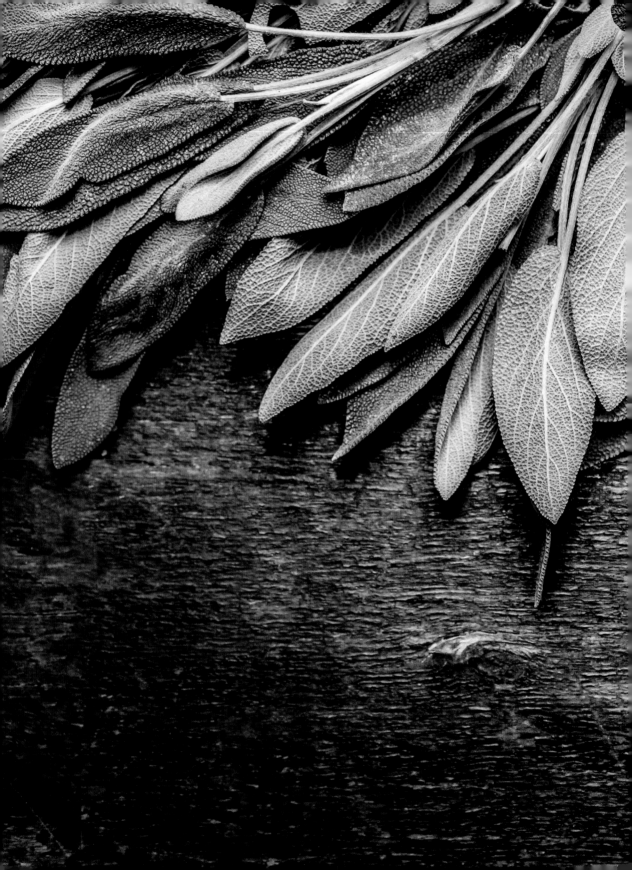

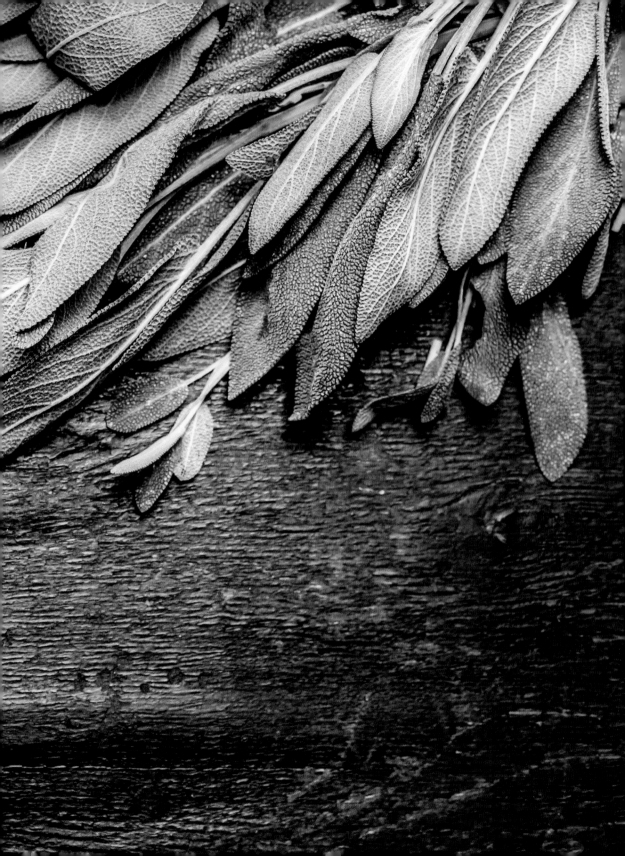

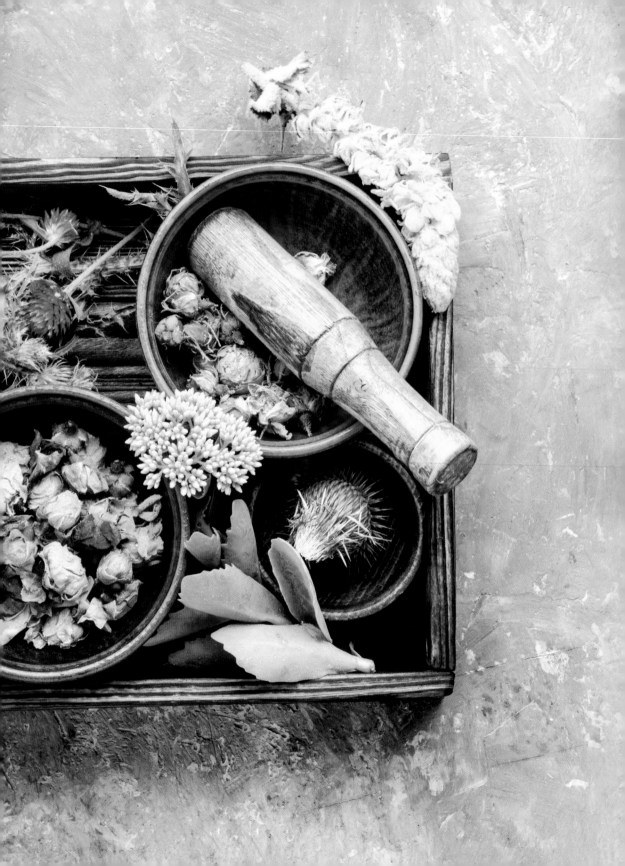

Glossary

Adaptogen: assists our physiological processes to cope with stressful stimuli.

Adrenal support: has a nurturing effect upon the adrenal system.

Adrenocorticomimetic: simulates the action of hormones of the adrenal cortex.

Anodyne: painkilling.

Anti-androgen: an agent that inhibits the actions or reduces the quantity of androgens (testosterone and dihydrotestosterone) in the system.

Anti-arrhythmic: agent utilised to suppress abnormal rhythms of the heart.

Anti-atheroma: agent utilised to remove accumulations of degenerative material from the inner layer of an artery wall, including cholesterol and plaque.

Anti-atherosclerotic: preventing lipid accumulation in arterial cells.

Anti-catarrhal: an agent utilised to help eliminate mucus from the sinuses and respiratory system.

Anticlastogenic: mitigates agents that cause damage to chromosomes.

Anticoagulant: inhibits blood-clotting mechanisms.

Antidyspeptic: counters indigestion.

Antiemetic: reduces the occurrence and intensity of nausea and vomiting.

Antihaemorrhagic: arrests bleeding.

Antihelmintic: prevents or eliminates parasitic worms.

Antihydrotic: agent which suppresses or prevents excessive perspiration.

Antihyperglycaemic: counters high spikes in blood sugar levels.

Antihyperlipidaemic: lowers levels of lipids in the blood.

Antimalarial: acts to prevent or cure malaria.

Antimutagenic: acts to inhibit or reduce the frequency of cellular mutation.

Anti-neuroinflammatory: inhibits or suppresses inflammation of the nervous tissue.

Anti-oestrogenic: inhibits the action or production of oestrogen.

Antioxidant: inhibits or slows oxidation damage to cells and other molecules.

Antiplatelet: acts to reduce platelet aggregation and inhibit thrombus formation.

Antiproliferative: suppresses or inhibits the spread of cancer cell lines.

Antipruritic: suppresses itch.

Antipyretic: Prevents or reduces temperature of fever.

Antiscrofulous: works to destroy or diminish scrofula (tuberculosis or TB-like bacteria) within the lymph nodes.

Antispasmodic: prevents or alleviates muscle spasms and cramps.

Anti-spirochetal: works to destroy or diminish activity of a group of spiral-shaped bacteria, including those implicated in Lyme disease, syphilis and yaws.

Anti-thrombotic: agent that reduces the formation of blood clots.

Anti-thyroid: acts as an antagonist upon thyroid hormones. Reduces excessive thyroid activity.

Antitussive: acts to suppress coughing.

Anxiolytic: mitigates or inhibits anxiety.

Aperient: stimulates appetite and exerts a mild laxative effect.

Aphrodisiac: stimulates sexual desire.

Astringent: causes contraction of the tissues, binding of wounds.

Bitter/bitter tonic: stimulates the gall bladder and improves digestion and natural detoxification.

Blood tonic: an agent that stimulates the production of more blood cells in the body.

Bronchial dilator: an agent that relaxes and expands bronchial muscles, opening air passages.

Capillary tonic: nurtures or protects capillaries.

Cardiotonic: nurtures or protects the heart.

Carminative: stomach muscle relaxant, promotes intestinal peristalsis, settles digestive system and alleviates flatulence and distension caused by gas.

Cathartic: a strong laxative.

Chemopreventive: acts to inhibit/halt the development of cancerous cells.

Chemoprotective: protects healthy tissue from the harmful/toxic effects of cancer therapies/drugs.

Cholagogue: stimulates the flow of bile from the liver.

Cholinergic: mimics the action of the neurotransmitter acetylcholine. Regulates nerve impulses.

Coronary vasodilator: improves blood supply to the heart.

Demulcent: acts to relieve inflammation or irritation.

Depurative: exerts purifying and detoxifying effects.

Diaphoretic: promotes perspiration and eliminates toxins through the skin.

Diuretic: promotes urination.

Emmenagogue: triggers menstruation, generally a stimulant/tonic to the female reproductive system.

Emollient: softens or soothes the skin.

Expectorant: removes mucus from respiratory system.

Febrifuge: reduces fever.

Galactagogue: promotes milk in nursing mothers.

Genitourinary support: nurtures or strengths the functions of the genital and urinary organs.

Haemostatic: stops haemorrhaging, arrests bleeding.

Hepatic: has an effect upon the liver.

Hepatoprotective: nurtures/supports the healthy functioning of the liver. Acts to prevent damage to the liver.

Hypocholesterolemic: exerts cholesterol-lowering effects.

Hypoglycaemic: exerts glucose-lowering effects.

Hypolipidaemic: exerts lipid-lowering effects.

Hypotensive: lowers blood pressure.

Hypnotic: promotes sleep.

Immunomodulatory: impacts upon the immune system to activate or suppress responses.

Insulinogenic: an agent that stimulates the production of insulin.

Lymphatic: relating to lymph or its secretion.

Mucoprotective: agent that acts to protect mucous membranes.

Nervine: exerts a calming or other beneficial effect upon the nervous system.

Neuroprotective: an agent active in the protection, recovery or regeneration of the nervous system.

Nootropic: agent utilised to improve cognitive functioning.

Oestrogenic: promotes the production of oestrogen or mimics the action of oestrogen.

Opioidergic: acts to modulate the opioid neuropeptide systems. Mostly utilised with pain management and neurotransmitter activation.

Peripheral circulatory stimulant: improves blood circulation to the extremities and finer capillaries.

Peripheral vasodilator: improves blood circulation to the extremities and finer capillaries.

Photoprotection: guards against UV damage.

Rubefacient: improves blood circulation to local area by drawing blood to skin surface.

Stomachic: strengthens or stimulates the stomach in relief of gastric disorders.

Styptic: externally applied to arrest bleeding by instigating clotting.

Testosterone modulation: modulates the production of testosterone.

Thermogenic: exerts a heating effect in the body via metabolic stimulation.

Tonic: generally a substance which engenders a sense of well-being to the body. Specific tonics tone and
    stimulate/strengthen specific bodily systems or related organs.

Uterine: acts upon the uterus in tonic or stimulant action.

Uterine tonic: relates to any herb with gynaecological demulcent, anti-inflammatory, antispasmodic or other
    properties beneficial to uterus functioning and health.

Vascular tonic: supports and tones the integrity of blood-vessel walls.

Vasodilator: widens blood vessels and may support a lowering of blood pressure.

Vasoprotective: is nutritive to the venous system and strengthens it against potential damage.

Vasorelaxant: reduces tension of blood-vessel walls.

Venotonic: has a tonic action upon the venous system.

Vulnerary: promotes healing of wounds. Arrests tissue degeneration.

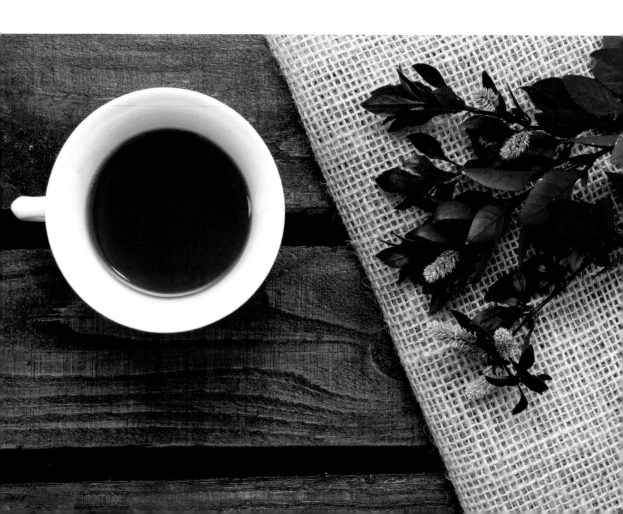

Bibliography

Akhondzadeh, S. *et al.*, 'Passionflower in the treatment of generalized anxiety: a pilot double-blind randomized controlled trial with oxazepam', *Journal of Clinical Pharmacy and Therapeutics,* Vol. 26, Issue 5, 2001, pp. 363–7

Amsterdam, J. D. *et al.*, 'A Randomized, Double-Blind, Placebo-Controlled Trial of Oral Matricaria recutita (Chamomile) Extract Therapy for Generalized Anxiety Disorder', *Journal of Clinical Psychopharma*, Vol. 29, Issue 4, 2009, pp. 378–82

Anderson, R. A. *et al.*, 'Isolation and characterization of polyphenol type-A polymers from cinnamon with insulin-like biological activity', *Diabetes Research and Clinical Practice*, Vol. 62, Issue 3, 2003, pp. 139–48

Apak, R. *et al.*, 'The cupric ion reducing antioxidant capacity and polyphenolic content of some herbal teas', *International Journal of Food Sciences and Nutrition,* Vol. 57, 2006, pp. 292–304

Applequist, W. J. and Moerman, D. E., 'Yarrow (*Achillea millefolium* L.): A neglected panacea? A review of ethnobotany, bioactivity and biomedical research', *Economic Botany*, Vol. 65, Issue 2, 2011, pp. 209–25

Aprotosoaie, A. C. *et al.*, 'Anethole and its role in Chronic Diseases', *Advances in Experimental Medicine and Biology*, Vol. 929, 2016, pp. 247–67

Awad, R. *et al.*, 'Effects of traditionally used anxiolytic botanicals on enzymes of the gamma-aminobutyric acid (GABA) system', *Canadian Journal of Physiology and Pharmacology*, Vol. 85, Issue 9, 2007, pp. 933–42

Barrett, B., 'Medicinal properties of *Echinacea*: a critical review', *Phytomedicine*, Vol. 10, 2003, pp. 66–86

Bates, S. H. *et al.*, 'Insulin-like effect of pinitol', *British Journal of Pharmacology*, Vol. 130, Issue 8, 2000, pp. 1944–8

Batta, S. K. and Santhakumari, G., 'Antifertility effect of *Ocimum Sanctum* and Hibiscus Rosa Sinensis', *Indian Journal of Medical Research*, Vol. 59, 1971, pp. 777–81

Belew, C., 'Herbs and the childbearing woman. Guidelines for midwives', *Journal of Nurse-Midwifery*, Vol. 44, 1999, pp. 231–52

Blumenthal, M. *et al.*, *The Complete German Commission E Monographs: Therapeutic Guide to Herbal Medicines* (The American Botanical Council, 1998)

Bracesco, N. *et al.*, 'Recent advances on *Ilex paraguariensis* research: mini-review', *Journal of Ethnopharmacology*, Vol. 136, Issue 3, 2011, pp. 378–84

Broadhurst, C. L. *et al.*, 'Insulin-like biological activity of culinary and medicinal plant aqueous extracts in vitro', *Journal of Agricultural and Food Chemistry*, Vol. 48, Issue 3, 2000, pp. 849–52

Buchbauer, G. *et al.*, 'Fragrance compounds and essential oils with sedative effects upon inhalation', *Journal of Pharmaceutical Science*, Vol. 82, 1993, pp. 660–4

Budzynska, K. *et al.*, 'Systematic Review of Breastfeeding and Herbs', *Breastfeeding Medicine*, Vol. 7, Issue 6, 2012, pp. 489–503

Bundy, R. *et al.*, 'Artichoke leaf extract reduces symptoms of irritable bowel syndrome and improves quality of life in otherwise healthy volunteers suffering from concomitant dyspepsia: A subset analysis', *Journal of Alternative and Complementary Medicine*, Vol. 10, 2004, pp. 4667–9

Carvajal-Zarrabal, O. *et al.*, '*Hibiscus sabdariffa* L., roselle calyx, from ethnobotany to pharmacology', *Journal of Experimental Pharmacology*, Vol. 28, Issue 4, 2012, pp. 25–39

Cetojevic-Simin, D. D., 'Antioxidative and antiproliferative activities of different horsetail (*Equisetum arvense* L.) extracts', *Journal of Medicinal Food*, Vol. 13, Issue 2, 2010, pp. 452–9

Chaoki, W. *et al.*, 'Citral inhibits cell proliferation and induces apoptosis and cell cycle arrest in MCF-7 cells', *Fundamental & Clinical Pharmacology*, Vol. 23, 2009, pp. 549–56

Chedraui, P. *et al.*, 'Effect of Trifolium pratense-derived isoflavones on the lipid profile of postmenopausal women with increased body mass index', *Gynecological Endocrinology*, Vol. 24, Issue 11, 2008, pp. 620–4

Chen, A. Y. and Chen, Y. C., 'A review of the dietary flavonoid kaempferol on human health and cancer chemoprevention', *Food Chemistry*, Vol. 138, Issue 4, 2013, pp. 2099–107

Clifford, L. J. *et al.*, 'Bioactivity of alkamides isolated from *Echinacea purpurea* (L.). Moench', *Phytomedicine*, Vol. 9, 2002, pp. 249–53

de la Garza, A. L. *et al.*, 'Natural inhibitors of pancreatic lipase as new players in obesity treatment', *Planta Medica*, Vol. 77, Issue 8, 2011, pp. 773–85

de Nysschen, A. M. *et al.*, 'The major phenolic compounds in the leaves of *Cyclopia* species (honeybush tea)', *Biochemical Systematics and Ecology,* Vol. 24, 1996, pp. 243–6

de Pascual-Teresa, S. *et al.*, 'Flavanols and anthocyanins in cardiovascular health: a review of current evidence', *International Journal of Molecular Science*, Vol. 11, 2010, pp. 1679–703

Diamond, B. J. *et al.*, 'Ginkgo biloba extract: mechanisms and clinical indications', *Archives of Physical Medicine and Rehabilitation*, Vol. 81, 2000, pp. 669–78

Du, G. J. *et al.*, 'Epigallocatechin Gallate (EGCG) Is the most effective cancer chemopreventive polyphenol in Green Tea', *Nutrients*, Vol. 4, 2012, pp. 1679–91

Duke, J. A., *Handbook of Phytochemical Constituents of GRAS Herbs and Other Economic Plants* (CRC Press, 1992)

Dulloo, A. *et al.*, 'Efficacy of a green tea extract rich in catechin polyphenols and caffeine in increasing 24 hour energy expenditure and fat oxidation in humans', *The American Journal of Clinical Nutrition*, Vol. 70, Issue 6, 1999, pp. 1040–5

Ekor, M., 'The growing use of herbal medicines: issues relating to adverse reactions and challenges in monitoring safety', *Frontiers in Pharmacology*, Vol. 4, 2013, p. 177

Fecka, I. and Turek, S., 'Determination of water-soluble polyphenolic compounds in commercial herbal teas from Lamiaceae: peppermint, melissa, and sage', *Journal of Agricultural and Food Chemistry*, Vol. 55, 2007, pp. 10908–17

Ferlemi, A. V. and Lamari, F. N., 'Berry Leaves: An Alternative Source of Bioactive Natural Products of Nutritional and Medicinal Value', *Antioxidants*, Vol. 5, Issue 2, 2016, p. 17

Gardiner, P., 'Complementary, Holistic, and Integrative Medicine: Chamomile', *Pediatrics in Review*, Vol. 28, 2007, pp. 16–18

González, R. *et al.*, 'Effects of flavonoids and other polyphenols on inflammation', *Critical Reviews in Food Science and Nutrition*, Vol. 51, Issue 4, 2011, pp. 331–62

Grant, P., 'Spearmint herbal tea has significant anti-androgen effects in polycystic ovarian syndrome. A randomized controlled trial', *Phytotherapy Research*, Vol. 24, Issue 2, 2010, pp. 186–8

Gray, A. M. *et al.*, 'The traditional plant treatment, *Sambucus nigra* (elder), exhibits insulin-like and insulin-releasing actions in vitro', *The Journal of Nutrition*, Vol. 130, Issue 1, 2010, pp. 15–20

Grundmann, O. *et al.*, 'Anxiolytic activity of a phytochemically characterized *Passiflora incarnata* extract is mediated via the GABAergic system', *Planta Medica*, Vol. 74; Issue 15, 2008, pp. 1769–73

Gudej, J. and Tomczyk, M., 'Determination of Flavonoids, Tannins, and Ellagic Acid in Leaves from Rubus L. Species', *Archives of Pharmacal Research*, Vol. 27, No 11, 2004, pp. 1114–19

Haskell, C. F. *et al.*, 'The effects of L-theanine, caffeine and their combination on cognition and mood', *Biological Psychology*, Vol. 77, No. 2, 2008, pp. 113–22

Hearst, C. *et al.*, 'Antibacterial activity of elder (*Sambucus nigra* L.) flower or berry against hospital pathogens', *Journal of Medicinal Plants Research*, Vol. 4, Issue 17, 2010, pp. 1805–9

Herrmann, M. *et al.*, 'Blackberry leaf extract: a multifunctional anti-aging active', *International Journal of Cosmetic Science*, Vol. 29, Issue 5, 2007, p. 411

Hidalgo, L. A. *et al.*, 'The effect of red clover isoflavones on menopausal symptoms, lipids and vaginal cytology in menopausal women: a randomized, double-blind, placebo-controlled study', *Gynecological Endocrinology*, Vol. 21, Issue 5, 2005, pp. 257–64

Huang, W. Y. *et al.*, 'Natural phenolic compounds from medicinal herbs and dietary plants: potential use for cancer prevention', *Nutrition and Cancer*, Vol. 62, Issue 1, 2010, pp. 1–20

Johnston, G. A., 'Flavonoid nutraceuticals and ionotropic receptors for the inhibitory neurotransmitter GABA', *Neurochemistry International*, Vol. 89, 2015, pp. 120–5

Kakuda, T., 'Neuroprotective effects of theanine and its preventative effects on cognitive dysfunction', *Pharmacological Research*, Vol. 64, No. 2, 2011, pp. 162–8

Kamara, B. *et al.*, 'Polyphenols from honeybush tea (*Cyclopia intermedia*)', *Journal of Agricultural and Food Chemistry*, Vol. 51, No. 13, 2003, pp. 3874–9

Katavic, P. L. *et al.*, 'Flavonoids as opioid receptor ligands: identification and preliminary structure-activity relationships', *Journal of Natural Products*, Vol. 70, Issue 8, 2007, pp. 1278–82

Kay, C. D. and Holub, B. J., 'The effect of wild blueberry (Vaccinium angustifolium) consumption on postprandial serum antioxidant status in human subjects', *British Journal of Nutrition*, Vol. 88, Issue 4, 2002, pp. 389–98

Kennedy, D. and Scholey, A., 'Ginseng: potential for the enhancement of cognitive performance and mood', *Pharmacology, Biochemistry, Behavior*, Vol. 75, 2003, pp. 687–700

Kennedy, D. O. *et al.*, 'Modulation of mood and cognitive performance following acute administration of single doses of *Melissa officinalis* (Lemon balm) with human CNS nicotinic and muscarinic receptor-binding properties', *Neuropsychopharmacology*, Vol. 28, Issue 10, 2003, pp. 1871–81

Khan, A. *et al.*, 'Cinnamon improves glucose and lipids of people with type 2 diabetes', *Diabetes Care*, Vol. 26, Issue 12, 2003, pp. 3215–18

Khan, A. and Gilani, A. H., 'Selective bronchodilatory effect of rooibos tea (*Aspalathus linearis*) and its flavonoid, chrysoeriol', *European Journal of Nutrition*, Vol. 45, 2006, pp. 463–9

Khasnavis, S. and Pahan, K., 'Sodium benzoate, a metabolite of cinnamon and a food additive, upregulates neuroprotective Parkinson disease protein DJ-1 in astrocytes and neurons', *Journal of Neuroimmune Pharmacology*, Vol. 7, Issue 2, 2012, pp. 424–35

Kianbakht, S. *et al.*, 'Antihyperlipidemic effects of Salvia officinalis L. leaf extract in patients with hyperlipidemia: A randomized double-blind placebo-controlled clinical trial', *Phytotherapy Research*, Vol. 25, 2011, pp. 1849–53

Konrad, L. *et al.*, 'Antiproliferative effect on human prostate cancer cells by a stinging nettle root (*Urtica dioica*) extract', *Planta Medica*, Vol. 66, Issue 1, 2000, pp. 44–7

Koulivand, P. H. *et al.*, 'Lavender and the Nervous System', *Evidence-Based Complementary and Alternative Medicine*, Vol. 2013, Article ID 681304

Ku, S. K. *et al.*, 'Orientin inhibits high glucose-induced vascular inflammation in vitro and in vivo', *Inflammation*, Vol. 37, Issue 6, 2014, pp. 2164–73

Ku, S. K. *et al.*, 'Aspalathin and Nothofagin from Rooibos (*Aspalathus linearis*) inhibits high glucose-induced inflammation in vitro and in vivo', *Inflammation*, Vol. 38, Issue 1, 2015, pp. 445–55

Kulisic, T. *et al.*, 'Antioxidant activity of aqueous tea infusions prepared from oregano, thyme and wild thyme', *Food Technology and Biotechnology*, Vol. 44, 2006, pp. 485–92

Kuroda, K. *et al.*, 'Sedative effects of the jasmine tea odor and (R)-(-)-linalool, one of its major odor components, on autonomic nerve activity and mood states', *European Journal of Applied Physiology*, Vol. 95, Issues 2–3, 2005, pp. 107–14

Lai, S. W. *et al.*, 'Novel Neuroprotective Effects of the Aqueous Extracts from *Verbena officinalis* Linn', *Neuropharmacology*, Vol. 50, Issue 6, 2006, pp. 641–50

Lee, R. J. and Cohen, N. A., 'Role of the bitter taste receptor T2R38 in upper respiratory infection and chronic rhinosinusitis', *Current Opinion in Allergy and Clinical Immunology*, Vol. 15, Issue 1, 2015, pp. 14–20

Lees, A., 'Dopamine agonists in Parkinson's disease: a look at apomorphine', *Fundamental & Clinical Pharmacology*, Vol. 7, Issues 3–4, 1993, pp. 121–8

Li, N., 'Platelet-lymphocyte cross-talk', *Journal of Leukocyte Biology*, Vol. 83, 2008, pp. 1069–78

Lin, C. C. *et al.*, 'Anti-inflammatory and radical scavenge effects of *Arctium lappa*', *The American Journal of Chinese Medicine*, Vol. 24, 1996, pp. 127–37

Lin, Y. *et al.*, 'Luteolin, a flavonoid with potential for cancer prevention and therapy', *Current Cancer Drug Targets*, Vol. 8, Issue 7, 2008, pp. 634–46

Liu, L.. *et al.*, 'Cinnamic acid: a natural product with potential use in cancer intervention', *International Journal of Cancer*, Vol. 28, Issue 62 (3), 1995, pp. 345–50

Liu, M. *et al.*, 'Pharmacological profile of xanthohumol, a prenylated flavonoid from hops (*Humulus lupulus*)', *Molecules*, Vol. 7, Issue 20 (1), 2015, pp. 754–79

Luo, Y. *et al.*, 'Antioxidant activity and phenolic compounds of 112 traditional Chinese medicinal plants associated with anticancer', *Life Science*, Vol. 74, 2004, pp. 2157–84

Makino, Y. *et al.*, 'Hastatoside and verbenalin are sleep-promoting components in *Verbena officinalis*', *Sleep and Biological Rhythms*, Vol. 7, Issue 3, 2009, pp. 211–17

Manayi, A. *et al.*, '*Echinacea purpurea*: Pharmacology, phytochemistry and analysis methods', *Pharmacognosy Reviews*, Vol. 9, Issue 17, 2015, pp. 63–72

Mármol, I. *et al.*, 'Therapeutic Applications of Rose Hips from Different *Rosa* Species', *International Journal of Molecular Sciences*, Vol. 18, Issue 6, 2017, p. 1137

Mayer, B. *et al.*, 'Gastroprotective constituents of *Salvia officinalis* L', *Fitoterapia*, Vol. 80, 2009, pp. 421–6

McCarthy, P., 'Safety of Herbal V Orthodox Drugs – one of the key issues under consideration by the IMB', *Irish Medical Times*, Vol. 35, No. 31, 2001 pp. 369–73

McKay, D. L. and Blumberg, J. B., 'A review of the bioactivity and potential health benefits of peppermint tea (*Mentha piperita* L.)', *Phytotherapy Research*, Vol. 20, 2006, pp. 619–33

Mimica-Dukic, N. *et al.*, 'Phenolic compounds in field horsetail (*Equisetum arvense L.*) as natural antioxidants', *Molecules*, Vol. 17, Issue 13 (7), 2008, pp. 1455–64

Miranda, C. L. *et al.*, 'Antiproliferative and cytotoxic effects of prenylated flavonoids from hops (*Humulus lupulus*) in human cancer cell lines', *Food and Chemical Toxicology*, Vol. 37, Issue 4, 1999, pp. 271–85

Mitjavila, M. T. and Moreno, J. J., 'The effects of polyphenols on oxidative stress and the arachidonic acid cascade. Implications for the prevention/treatment of high prevalence diseases', *Biochemical Pharmacology*, Vol. 84, 2012, pp. 1113–22

Morton, J. F., 'Rooibos tea, *Aspalathus linearis*, a caffeineless, low-tannin beverage', *Economic Botany*, Vol. 37, 1983, pp. 164–73

Mozaffari-Khosravi, H. *et al.*, 'Effects of sour tea (*Hibiscus sabdariffa*) on lipid profile and lipoproteins in patients with type II diabetes', *The Journal of Alternative and Complementary Medicine*, Vol. 15, Issue 8, 2009, pp. 899–903

Osakabe, N. *et al.*, 'Anti-inflammatory and anti-allergic effect of rosmarinic acid (RA); inhibition of seasonal allergic rhinoconjunctivitis (SAR) and its mechanism', *Biofactors*, Vol. 21, Issues 1–4, 2004, pp. 127–31

Ovadje, P. *et al.*, 'Dandelion root extract affects colorectal cancer proliferation and survival through the activation of multiple death signalling pathways', *Oncotarget*, Vol. 7, Issue 45, 2016, pp. 73080–100

Pascual, M. E. *et al.*, 'Lippia: Traditional uses, chemistry and pharmacology: A review', *Journal of Ethnopharmacology*, Vol. 76, Issue 3, 2001, pp. 201–14

Phillips, S. *et al.*, '*Zingiber officinale* (ginger) – an antiemetic for day case surgery', *Anaesthesia*, Vol. 48, Issue 8, 1993, pp. 715–17

Pleschka, S. *et al.*, 'Anti-viral properties and mode of action of standardized Echinacea purpurea extract against highly pathogenic avian influenza virus (H5N1, H7N7) and swine-origin H1N1 (S-OIV)', *Virology Journal*, Vol. 6, 2009, p. 197

Pompei, R. *et al.*, 'Glycyrrhizic acid inhibits virus growth and inactivates virus particles', *Nature*, Vol. 281 (5733), 1979, pp. 689–90

Puangpraphant, S. *et al.*, 'Dicaffeoylquinic acids in Yerba mate (*Ilex paraguariensis* St. Hilaire) inhibit NFKB nucleus translocation in macrophages and induce apoptosis by activating caspases 8 and 3 in human colon cancer cells', *Molecular Nutrition and Food Research*, Vol. 55, Issue 10, 2001, pp. 1509–22

Roschek, B. *et al.*, 'Elderberry flavonoids bind to and prevent H1N1 infection in vitro', *Phytochemistry*, Vol. 70, 2009, pp. 1255–61

Sa, C. M. *et al.*, 'Sage tea drinking improves lipid profile and antioxidant defences in humans', *International Journal of Molecular Science*, Vol. 10, 2009, pp. 3937–50

Safarinejad, M. R., '*Urtica dioica* for treatment of benign prostatic hyperplasia: a prospective, randomized, double-blind, placebo-controlled, crossover study', *Journal of Herbal Pharmacotherapy*, Vol. 5, Issue 4, 2005, pp. 1–11

Santos, M. *et al.*, 'An Aqueous Extract of Valerian Influences Transport of GABA in Synaptosomes', *Planta Medica*, Vol. 60, 1994, pp. 278–9

Schutz, K. *et al.*, 'Taraxacum – a review on its phytochemical and pharmacological profile', *Journal of Ethnopharmacology*, Vol. 107, Issue 3, 2006, pp. 313–23

Sehdev, V. *et al.*, 'Biochanin A Modulates Cell Viability, Invasion, and Growth Promoting Signalling Pathways in HER-2-Positive Breast Cancer Cells', *Journal of Oncology*, 2009, article ID: 121458

Semwal, R. B. *et al.*, 'Gingerols and shogaols: Important nutraceutical principles from ginger', *Phytochemistry*, Vol. 117, 2015, pp. 554–68

Shahidi, F., 'Antioxidants in food and food antioxidants', *Food/Nahrung*, Vol. 44, 2000, pp. 158–63

Shankar, E. *et al.*, 'Plant flavone apigenin: An emerging anticancer agent', *Current Pharmacology Reports*, Vol. 3, Issue 6, 2017, pp. 423–46

Stephens, F. O., 'Phytoestrogens and prostate cancer: possible preventive role', *The Medical Journal of Australia*, Vol. 167, 1997, pp. 138–40

Theoharides, T. C. *et al.*, 'Brain "fog", inflammation and obesity: key aspects of neuropsychiatric disorders improved by luteolin', *Frontiers in Neuroscience*, Vol. 9, 2015, p. 225

Ukiya, M. *et al.*, 'Constituents of Compositae plants III. Anti-tumor promoting effects and cytotoxic activity against human cancer cell lines of triterpene diols and triols from edible chrysanthemum flowers', *Cancer Letters*, Vol. 177, Issue 1, 2002, pp. 7–12

Venè, R. *et al.*, 'Xanthohumol impairs human prostate cancer cell growth and invasion and diminishes the incidence and progression of advanced tumors in TRAMP mice', *Molecular Medicine*, Vol. 18, 2012, pp. 1292–1302

Viola, H. *et al.*, 'Isolation of pharmacologically active benzodiazepine receptor ligands from *Tilia tomentose* (Tiliaceae)', *Journal of Ethnopharmacology*, Vol. 44, 1994, pp. 47–53

Vishnuvathan, V. J. *et al.*, 'Medicinal Uses of Formononetin – a review', *The Journal of Ethnobiology and Traditional Medicine*, Vol. 126, 2016, pp. 1197–209

World Health Organization, Programme on Traditional Medicine. *Guidelines for the Assessment of Herbal Medicines* (Geneva, WHO, 1991)

World Health Organization, *Research Guidelines for Evaluating the Safety and Efficacy of Herbal Medicines* (Manila, Regional Office for the Western Pacific, 1993)

World Health Organization, *Guidelines for the Appropriate Use of Herbal Medicines* (Manila, Regional Office for the Western Pacific, 1998)

Xu, J. G., *et al.*, 'Antioxidant and DNA-Protective Activities of Chlorogenic Acid Isomers', *Journal of Agricultural and Food Chemistry*, Vol. 60, 2012, pp. 11625–30

Xu, L. *et al.*, 'Apigenin, a dietary flavonoid, sensitizes human T cells for activation-induced cell death by inhibiting PKB/Akt and NF-kappaB activation pathway', *Immunology Letters*, Vol. 121, Issue 1, 2008, pp. 74–83

Yan, X. *et al.*, 'Apigenin in cancer therapy: anti-cancer effects and mechanisms of action', *Cell & Bioscience,* Vol. 7, 2017, p. 50

Yi, W. *et al.*, 'Phenolic compounds from blueberries can inhibit colon cancer cell proliferation and induce apoptosis', *Journal of Agricultural and Food Chemistry*, Vol. 53, Issue 18, 2005, pp. 7320–9

Yoshimaru, T. *et al.*, 'Xanthohumol suppresses oestrogen-signalling in breast cancer through the inhibition of BIG3-PHB2 interactions', *Scientific Reports,* Vol. 4, 2014, p. 7355

Zhang, L. *et al.*, 'Ginkgo biloba Extract for Patients with Early Diabetic Nephropathy: A Systematic Review', *Evidence-Based Complementary and Alternative Medicine*, 2013, p. 689142

Index

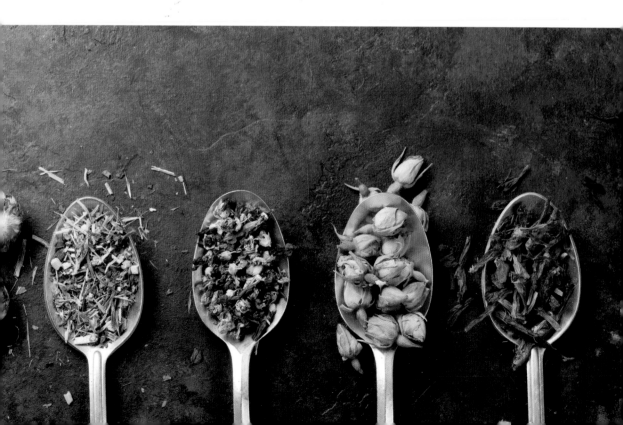